My Home Pharmacy

How Foods and Herbs Can Be Your Medicine

Tracy Gibbs, PhD

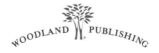

WOODLAND PUBLISHING

For permissions, ordering information, or bulk quantity discounts, contact: Woodland Publishing, Salt Lake City, UT

Visit our website: www.woodlandpublishing.com
Toll-free number (800) 777-BOOK

Note: The information in this book is for educational purposes only and is not recommended as a means of diagnosing or treating an illness. All matters concerning physical and mental health should be supervised by a health practitioner knowledgeable in treating that particular condition. Neither the publisher nor the authors directly or indirectly dispense medical advice, nor do they prescribe any remedies or assume any responsibility for those who choose to treat themselves.

ISBN: 978-1-58054-149-7

Printed in the United States of America

A book that sets the standard for others to follow does not come around very often. Tracy has accomplished a work that not only is as simple to understand as a common cookbook, but that also advances the understanding of even the most educated herbalists and doctors. His common-sense science will help all of us who are doctors remember why we wanted to become doctors in the first place.

–Dr. J. Frederic Templeman, MD

Recently there has been a renewed interest by the medical profession into the beneficial effects of natural products and herbs for chronic disease and the prevention thereof. It is estimated that over 80 percent of the world's population relies heavily on natural plant products as medicines and drugs. Half of the top 50 drugs sold in European pharmacies are based on or derived from natural herbs. Perhaps the U.S. market can learn something from Tracy's book. Despite much of our scientific research into natural herbs, our knowledge in how to actually use them on patients remains inadequate. Tracy gives us a guidebook to follow, and perhaps through using his formulas we will come to a better understanding of why and how these "food medicines" really work.

–Dr. Yi-Zhun Zhu, MD
(Dean of Pharmacology, Singapore National University)

Contents

Preface

As recently as 50 years ago, most households had a small folder, a binder, a 3-inch by 5-inch card holder or a family "secret recipe" book. This heirloom contained information similar to what you will find in this book. Such family recipes were usually passed down from parent to child, generation after generation. When someone became sick, this collected wisdom was put to use with a lot of care and love.

As children, many of us may have experienced the use of such recipes when our own mothers or grandmothers created special brews and coaxed us into drinking some nasty-tasting concoction. Whether they called it birch bark tea, sage tea, firewater, "Aunt Betty's Revenge" or whatever else, you may remember ingesting a foul-smelling remedy while you lay sick in bed. And those memories are hard to erase, because even though you suffered and likely complained during the brew's administration, you probably also can't deny that the next day you felt better.

Many family heirloom recipe books have disappeared in the last few decades. Many people have lost this knowledge or did not pass it on due to a series of events that took place within the last century. If you are among the millions of people to whom this information has been lost, don't worry; this book was written just for you. You can use it as your starting point. From here you can add your own notes and adjustments as you begin to understand how the body works. This book will help you begin to take responsibility for your health and the health of your loved ones. After all, only you can take responsibility for your own health. And if you have children, only a parent can make sure your little ones receive the care they need and deserve.

Acknowledgements

Many people have sprinkled the seeds of inspiration in my life. Though many of these seeds landed on the rocky soil of my heart, many more eventually sprouted, leading to the bountiful harvest that fills my life today. Among those I must mention is my grandmother, Lottie Gibbs, from Moreland, Idaho. Grandma Gibbs spent many days with me as a child, and I can still recall her use of herbs to fix everything from a bad case of strep throat to bee stings and high fevers.

I must also thank my mother, Nancy Gibbs, who taught me about the use of herbs through experimentation on my siblings and me. I recall a time when both my mother and I were sick and drank some birch bark tea. We gagged while we sipped it down, but sure enough we were better by the next morning. My father, Ronald Gibbs, also deserves special credit for his patience and trust in me.

Special thanks go to Tosha Arnout, who is an expert at formulating lotions and creams and who assisted me where my knowledge was insufficient. Thanks, too, to Kat (Kathryn) Gille, who has a natural ability to discover the words that I wanted to say but could not find.

Finally I must thank my three children, Tyler, Dylan and Nathan. They have been the "guinea pigs" for many of my home remedies. They have also patiently endured my countless lectures on why candy is not good for them. Their love and respect has been worth more than all the gold in the world.

Old vs. New: A History of Medicine

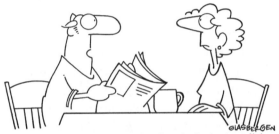

"Many people believe that laughter is the best medicine,
so the government has declared a ban on all laughing
until further studies can be done."

When asked whether the use of herbs can help an ailment or disease, many doctors may scoff and cite harmful side effects while declaring herbs "out of date" or old-fashioned, even though many people now use herbs on a regular basis. I always ask those who scoff to keep an open mind. You should never criticize something until you have tried it yourself, studied it in depth or heard the firsthand experience of someone who has put it to use. And yet many people mock the idea that "natural remedies" can be as (or more) effective than expensive pharmaceutical medications sold in pharmacies.

There is a simple explanation for this skepticism. *Until very recently, science was quite behind the times.* In the last 20 years, science has partially caught up with herbal medicine. Some people reading this might ask, "Don't you mean that herbal medicine is outdated or behind the times?" No, I don't. Here are some examples.

In her 1999 book, *An Enumeration of Chinese Materia Medica,* Shiu-ying Hu reports that in a Chinese document dating back to around 3000 BC, a physician diagnosed a patient with a goiter. The physician recommended the patient eat a strict diet of seaweed, and the patient was cured within a few weeks. Yet it was not until 1860 (4,860 years later) that modern science discovered that iodine (found in seaweed) is an essential nutrient. Today, iodine is used to treat goiters.

Here's another example: According to an article by Paul Carrick in *Clinical Medical Ethics* in 2001, anemia was first documented as a disease around 400 BC in both Greek and Egyptian texts. The common treatment was to have the patient drink water that had been used to cool hot iron as it was shaped in a blacksmith's shop. And yet modern science did not consider the mineral iron to be essential to the human body until the mid-1700s (over 2,000 years later).

Another example: Greek physician Hippocrates, who lived in the fifth and fourth centuries BC, commonly fed patients chicken and goat livers to cure night blindness, an inability to see in dim light caused by a vitamin A deficiency. The active compound in these livers (vitamin A) was not discovered until 1913 (about 2,300 years later).

A final example: in his 2003 book *Scurvy: How a Surgeon, a Mariner, and a Gentleman Solved the Greatest Medical Mystery of the Age of Sail*, Stephen R. Bown reports that scurvy plagued every navy from 2500 BC to the 1700s AD. James Lind, a British naval surgeon in the mid-18th century, discovered that lemons and limes prevented the degenerating effects of this disease. It took science over 200 years to catch up to Lind's discovery, but eventually scientists found that a lack of vitamin C caused scurvy. Vitamin C is found abundantly in citrus fruits like lemons and limes.

Frequently, knowing that certain compounds are effective treatments for diseases, scientists form theories and conduct various experiments to discover why these plant materials work in the human body the way they do.

Now you know why I write that science has finally begun to catch up with herbal medicine. It has only been in the last 15–20 years that science has discovered hundreds of unique compounds in plants that hold the keys to treating many degenerative conditions, including heart disease, cancer and diabetes. These active compounds, known as *phytochemicals*, contain both nutritional and medicinal value. Hundreds more phytochemicals have been discovered but their purposes or functions are still unknown. Perhaps someday soon the cures for multiple sclerosis, lupus, arthritis and other debilitating diseases will be discovered within untested compounds found in common plants.

Today, many doctors agree that much evidence supports the use of herbs in both healing and preventing illnesses, but conventional doctors often still do not know how to use them.

Until recently, doctors who graduated from allopathic medical schools were not required to take classes in herbs, plant-based drugs or even nutrition basics. Though herbs are still not studied in depth, many medical schools now mention them and new physicians are often much more open-minded and are slowly becoming better trained. Some doctors, however, still scoff at those who use herbs as medicine. Many doctors believe that if you can't explain why something works, it might be dangerous and it is best not to use it.

This focus on scientific evidence made the 1960s, '70s and '80s a "golden age" of allopathic medicine (those who practice *allopathic medicine* use only drugs or surgery that are based on scientific evidence to combat disease, as opposed to *naturopathic medicine* practitioners, who use historically established remedies found in nature). During these years, many medical practitioners turned away from the old time-tested and proven ways that allowed the body to heal itself and switched to "instant gratification" drugs and over-the-counter (OTC) drugs. The American lifestyle demanded an instant fix. "We don't have time to miss work for a day or two" demanded the public. Many people switched to new drugs that television commercials and doctors promised would provide simple, easy and effective cures for common ailments.

During the 1950s, '60s and '70s, allopathic physicians generally ignored the use of herbs. In the 1980s, many doctors labeled the use of herbs as "unpredictable and dangerous." Then, in the 1990s, as new testing methods began to add evidence to the benefits of herbs, allopathic physicians started using a new name for the use of herbs in healing: "alternative medicine." To those of us who had always used herbs, the name was somewhat comical and even absurd because we viewed prescription drugs as the newcomers and therefore the true "alternative." Even though herbs have been used as medicine for hundreds and even thousands of years, and even though herbs are still commonly used by over 80 percent of the world's population, the term "alternative medicine" became the common name for herbal medicine in the United States.

The popularity of herbs as medicine continues to grow as people try herbal remedies and like the results! The high prices and high risk of prescription drugs have also motivated the expanded use of safer, more traditional therapies. Currently, as new physicians are being educated on the use of herbs as medicine, a new type of practitioner is becoming more common. Doctors who both practice allopathic medicine and use herbal remedies sometimes refer to themselves as "complementary physicians" and to their methods as "complementary medicine."

It took only 50 years from when most people stopped using herbs to their reintroduction into the halls of medicine with a new name. Have we seen the end of changes in the pharmaceutical world? Not by a long shot. The entire pharmaceutical industry has a short history of only about 90 years. Homeopathy (a medical practice that treats diseases using small doses of a remedy that would cause symptoms of that disease in larger doses) has a much longer history of over 200 years. Pharmacognosy (the study of the medicinal use of plants) has a documented history in many countries dating back to the origins of each new culture.

According to Joost Visser in the book *Complementary Medicine and the European Community*, several modern countries such as Finland, Germany and Norway have more licensed homeopathic physicians than allopathic physicians. In Asia, allopathic Western medicine is truly the alternative method. Many of the older generations in Asia continue to visit herbal medicine doctors whenever they are faced with an ailment they can't take care of themselves. Does the rest of the world know something that Americans do not? Should we too have access to "alternative" forms of medicine that are mainstream in the rest of the world?

The Rise of the Prescription Drug

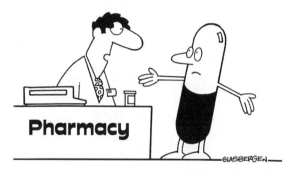

Copyright 2002 by Randy Glasbergen.
www.glasbergen.com

GLASBERGEN

"Well there's a side effect I haven't seen before."

Allopathic medicine has been credited with adding several years to the average human lifespan. Many practitioners in the herbal industry don't believe this information, but it is true. However, a common misconception regarding this statistic is that the *prescription drug industry* aided in this extension of lifespan. That is certainly not true. Allopathic medicine, independent of the prescription drug industry, plays an integral role in trauma treatment and saves thousands of people from trauma-related deaths each day.

Prior to World War II (1939–1945), for example, the average life-span of the American male was very low—due not to degenerative diseases, but to the high number of trauma-related deaths. War, work-related accidents and common infections were the major causes of death among *middle-aged* people near the turn of the 20th century. Several studies have shown that if a male lived past the age of 47 years in that era, he would most likely live well into his 80s. Advancements in trauma treatment and the proper sterilizing of hospital environments have lengthened the average lifespan—and both can be attributed to allopathic medicine.

Over the last 60 years, the major causes of death have slowly changed from trauma-related incidents to degenerative diseases. However, a new cause of death has crept up the scales: *medical care–related deaths*. According to an article published in the *Journal of the American Medical Association*, of the 225,000 people who die every year from medical care, 106,000 die from the normal use of prescription drugs while another 7,000 die from medication errors. An additional 80,000 die from hospital-borne infections that could have been prevented if not for the overuse of antibiotics. These statistics are incredible but true and, not surprisingly, are not well publicized.

During the past 40 years, the prescription drug industry has been expanding its markets to include the treatment of degenerative disease with more drugs, thus increasing its market share. Companies within this industry have effectively included allopathic doctors as "sales agents," in their marketing campaigns, but these new drugs have accomplished very little in curing any degenerative disease. Most of the products of the pharmaceutical drug industry target the temporary treatment or relief of a disease symptom instead of its permanent cure or prevention. Most degenerative diseases take years to develop within the body and cannot be cured in days or hours. However, since our society demands instant fixes, the drug industry produces drugs that fulfill our demand to take away the symptoms while doing little to cure the underlying disease. Americans spend billions of dollars every year on prescription drugs that cover up the symptoms of ailments such as cancer, diabetes, heart disease, Alzheimer's disease and arthritis, without curing anything.

Recently, prescription drug companies have started another new marketing campaign that pretends to focus on a new term called "preventative care." To the herbal industry, this term would mean strengthening the immune system, eating properly, breathing fresh air, drinking clean water and cultivating a low-stress environment. To the prescription drug industry, however, preventative care means spending billions of dollars on "early diagnostic equipment" to find problems earlier on, so you begin taking a prescription drug sooner.

Please don't misunderstand; allopathic medicine can save lives. If you have a trauma incident (such as a broken leg), go to an allopathic doctor, not your local herbalist. If your appendix bursts, go to the emergency room at a local hospital. If you are having a stroke or are in a car accident, call an ambulance! If you have a degenerative condition, however, what can an allopathic doctor do? Probably nothing! An herbalist, on the other hand, can rely on centuries and even millennia of traditional medical knowledge to find a natural way to enable the body to heal itself. History has shown that degenerative conditions are best treated and cured by herbs and dietary changes, not prescription drug intervention.

Yet seeking alternative care is against the law in many cases. In most states, it has become illegal for an herbalist to treat any condition, even a common cough. The technical language in the law books of most states makes it illegal for you to even put a bandage on a cut on your child's finger—you could be arrested for practicing medicine without a license. For example, the law in my home state of Utah states that anyone who diagnoses, advises, recommends, administers or dispenses a drug, medicine or treatment of *any* kind for *any* injury or illness is considered to be practicing medicine.

In other words, under current Utah state law, you could be arrested if you advised your grandmother to drink a glass of grape juice for her sore throat. You could be tried and convicted of a felony for applying an antibiotic cream on the skinned knee of your son or daughter. Would this ever really happen? I would hope not, but the law says it can. Your rights and freedom over your own body have been violated by lawmakers and some government-sponsored administrations. I believe individuals should always be allowed to choose for themselves the medical treatment for their own bodies.

We should all have the right to choose our own medical treatment. The laws regarding the practice of medicine must be re-evaluated and modified to include traditionally safe remedies as acceptable treatments that can be administered by anyone of your choosing. As the primary caregivers for their families, mothers and fathers should have every legal right and protection to choose medical treatments for their children.

In order to make wise health choices, however, we must educate ourselves in the basics of bodily functions and the uses of herbs and drugs. We cannot assume that all self-proclaimed herb experts will know how to help us any more than we can assume that anyone with a PhD or MD at the end of his or her name will know.

In 2003, the nationally televised case of 12-year-old Utah resident Parker Jensen caught the attention of many alternative medicine advocates as a classic example of what could happen if we do not re-evaluate existing laws. Parker was diagnosed with a type of oral cancer in 2003. His father, Daren Jensen, researched his son's particular type of oral cancer and determined that chemotherapy was not the best option. Jensen sought alternative care against the oncologist's recommendations. The oncologist sought state intervention and a judge ordered that Parker start chemotherapy by a certain date. When Parker's parents drove him to Idaho for alternative treatments instead, the judge ordered that Parker be placed in state protective custody. Parker's father was arrested in Idaho and charged with kidnapping, although these charges were later dropped. Despite the legal wranglings, Parker was not forced to undergo chemotherapy and the alternative treatments his parent sought were effective. Parker's cancer went into remission using alternative methods, as proven by several biopsies that were later presented as evidence to the court and the media.

In this case, Daren and Barbara Jensen did everything right. They researched their options and studied the information presented to them. They showed genuine care and interest in their son, and they sought professional help from both allopathic and alternative practitioners. They are a supreme example of how to act when illness befalls you or a loved one. When you are in need of professional advice regarding proper care for your body, you should seek help from both herbalists and allopathic physicians. They both will have answers and ideas that can help you.

However, if you need to ask a professional's opinion on the use of an herb, find a professional who knows about the use of herbs. Don't just assume that an allopathic doctor will know. Many physicians don't know about herbs and alternative medical treatments because they simply have not received training in these subjects.

An allopathic physician once told me that asking him about the use of herbs was like asking an auto mechanic to pick the high-trading stock of the day. Medical doctors lack the fundamental knowledge you are seeking. How can they answer questions about the use of vitamin A or chamomile? If you asked an allopathic doctor about digitoxin (a common drug to treat heart conditions), for example, I bet he or she could tell you all about its use, but he or she probably wouldn't know that it originated from a common herb known as foxglove. How about aspirin? Aspirin is a synthesized version of salicin, found mostly in white willow bark. Morphine comes from opium derived from poppies, quinine from cinchona bark, statins are found in red yeast rice, etc. These herbal remedies have been time tested and used by millions of people worldwide. Though science couldn't explain why they worked until recently, some people have spent their entire lives studying the use of these herbs, and they know which herb can best help you.

On the other hand, why would you go see an herbalist for acute appendicitis or a broken arm or leg? They have never been trained to perform complex operations or to set a bone. I know of a Nevada family that abhors allopathic doctors so much, when their 10-year-old son broke his arm, the mother set it herself and applied a plaster cast. Nine months later the son's arm was severely deformed. He still wore the cast for support and had almost no muscle mass due to atrophy from underuse. Herbal medicine and allopathic medicine are companions, and both deserve to be respected and treated as equal sciences.

It is amazing to me how much we disregard our own cultural heritage and how little knowledge we have of the unique and amazing plants that grow in our own backyards. Outspoken environmentalists, who are so passionate about saving endangered rain forests in faraway countries using the "potential loss of medicinal discoveries" as one rationale, ignore the common medicinal properties of North American species. North American medicinal plants are used extensively and constitute a huge market in Europe. Of the 232 entries in the *British Herbal Pharmacopoeia* (an authoritative source of information about pharmaceutical substances and medicinal products), 73 (over 30 percent) are indigenous to North America. According to the United States Department of Agriculture (USDA), medicinal plants also constitute a large portion of plant exports from the U.S. to the European Union.

It is my hope that Americans will find their roots again and that patience and understanding will dominate our decision-making process. Doctors everywhere should limit the use of prescription drugs to an absolute "as needed" basis and become more educated on subjects such as food and nutrition in relation to disease.

Many doctors reject the idea that natural treatments can be effective. Dr. Stephen Barrett, the outspoken, anti-alternative medicine writer and founder of Quackwatch.org[SM] goes so far as to say, "There is no logical reason to believe that dietary strategies can cure cancer. The idea that a natural diet can do so is absurd." Has Dr. Barrett forgotten the basic physiological mechanisms of the body's ability to heal itself if given the proper time and nutrients? This type of close-minded, extremely biased method of thought needs to be eliminated. Have Americans come to rely on pharmaceutical drugs and man-made interventions so completely that we have forgotten the basic elements that make up our own bodies? We have all learned that we need to keep active, moderate our diets, reduce our empty caloric intake and limit or avoid chemicals and drugs that are harmful to the body. If we know how to become healthy, then it is time we do it and begin to take responsibility for our own health instead of relying on the pharmaceutical, insurance or medical industries to make the decisions for us.

History of Herbs as Medicine

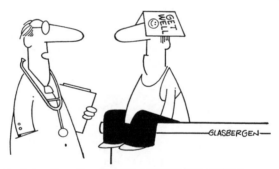

"That's all the alternative medicine your HMO will pay for."

Western herbology derives most of its roots from the ancient healing arts of Egypt. Most of the methods used by herbalists today—including herbal teas, hydrotherapy, exercise, diet and other forms of natural healing—were well documented in Egyptian writings. According to David Hoffman in *The Information Source Book of Herbal Medicine*, in around 500

BC, Greek scholars translated many Egyptian documents and not only recorded but put into practice many such therapies. During the "golden age" of herbology (from 200 BC to 200 AD), physicians began to classify herbs into categories according to their healing properties. Documents and uses cited by Greek physicians Dioscorides (40–90 AD) and Galen (129–200 AD) in the first and second centuries AD are still used widely in herbal books today and represent the foundation for all modern pharmacopoeias.

During the 12 centuries immediately following this golden age, many of the medicinal uses of these plants were forgotten or banned. Some well-known remedies were carried away into the Arab world after the Arabs intermingled with the Crusaders, and many were lost when the Roman Catholic Church discouraged them, claiming that the use of herbs constituted witchcraft or at least a lack of faith in God's power to heal.

Not until the early 18th century did herbal medicine again find a place in Western civilization. At that time, Carl Linné (1707–1778), the great Swedish botanist, compiled an international classification of plant names, which allowed plants all over the globe to be properly documented and compared for reference. Meanwhile, the expansive Portuguese, Spanish and British trade movements reawakened interest in botanical research, and investigations around the world led to the discovery and classification of hundreds of new medicinal plants. The revival of Western herbology went forward at full steam all over Europe and especially in the newly formed United States of America.

In the early days of the United States, home herbal remedies were more the rule than the exception. Many American medical textbooks that date back to the 1800s are full of references to plants and their uses. *The Old Farmer's Almanac,* the oldest continuously published periodical in the U.S., has published trusted home herbal remedies for a myriad of diseases and ailments since 1792. Most early physicians, including some of the country's founding fathers, used medicinal plants when treating ailments. Thomas Jefferson referenced unregulated remedies when he was addressing the issue of whether a federal commission should be established to regulate food consumption in the newly formed United States. In *Notes on the State of Virginia,* Jefferson said, "If the people let the government decide what foods they should eat *and what medicines they should take,* their bodies would soon be in as sorry a state as the souls of those of individuals who live under the suppressing hand of tyranny" (emphasis added). I wonder what ol' Tom would say if he saw the U.S. Food and Drug Administration (FDA) and its policies on drug approval methods. Truly we have seen his prophecy fulfilled as the FDA tells us what foods and herbs we can and can't use, and compare the current state of health in the United States with that of other developed countries.

However, the downfall of herbal medicine in the United States was caused not by religious crusades or unpopularity but by capitalism and greed. Capitalism, the foundation of the economy of the United States, is praised worldwide and is a great economic policy. However, combined with aggressive greed and bad politics, it can work against the public good. Such is the case with the herbal medicine industry in the United States. Between the years of 1890 and 1950, a series of events changed American medicine. During this time, start-up pharmaceutical companies backed by large investors began using political lobbies and the media to create laws that would essentially eliminate natural medicine by making the use of natural remedies illegal—all in the name of public safety.

Such policies ushered in the age of patent medicine and, consequently, the domination of the drug industry by corporate giants. Simply put, because a natural remedy cannot be patented, and therefore market domination cannot occur, such a remedy is of no interest to pharmaceutical giants. By making natural remedies illegal, or at least by convincing the public to perceive them as unsafe, pharmaceutical companies can gain 100 percent of the market share. Capitalism and greed have created a market in which the best remedy can easily be ousted in favor of the most profitable one. By the 1960s, prescription medicine was considered the norm instead of the alternative—both in the United States and in many other countries influenced by the United States.

Food-Medicine, Medicine-Food?

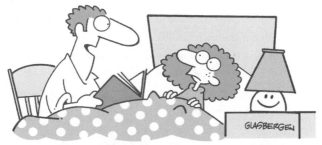

"First Goldilocks ate Papa Bear's porridge, then she ate Momma Bear's porridge, then she ate Baby Bear's porridge...and her cholesterol dropped 14 points!"

Herbal medicine is basically any natural plant material that is used for the benefit or treatment of an ailment in both humans and animals. What many people do not realize is that many "herbal remedies" are foods that you and I consume every day.

As stated before, the origin of herbal medicine dates back

to the beginning of time. Many people have asked, "How did ancient people know which herb to use for which disorder? They didn't have the science or the understanding of the human body we now have, so how did they know?" It's an interesting question and one that I also asked several years back. Specifically, I wondered how ancient Japanese people knew that they should eat wasabi (green horseradish) with sushi. If not prepared properly, sushi can contain a large amount of bacteria. Wasabi not only has antiseptic properties but also has a detoxifying effect in the liver. How did the ancient Japanese people know this?

And how did the ancient Saxons know to eat a similar herb, horseradish, with cured, uncooked beef and pork? What about Italian people, who ate seafood with oregano or garlic, both of which contain powerful antibiotic properties? Are these things just coincidence, or did ancient people hold an intuition that we have lost in modern times?

I believe the answer is quite simple. It is my opinion and observation that perhaps in the past, people were more in tune with the Earth, and, because science did not dominate their lives and minds, they were more humble and more willing to *ask* for help . . . and nature answered!

During my travels for both work and education, I have lived with indigenous peoples of many cultures. Several times the local "medicine man" has talked about how he "speaks" with the forest when problems arise.

Though to a Western-trained physician, this may sound absurd, at one time every culture throughout the world had holy men who spoke with nature. I believe that over time, knowledge thus obtained became tradition and tradition eventually became part of culture. My theory is that as humans gained more and more wisdom in the use of plants, tribal holy men developed, recorded and practiced standardized treatments. As tribal expansion caused the mixing of cultures, crafts and medicinal remedies, commonalities were found, resulting in the standardization of certain treatments.

In *An Enumeration of Chinese Materia Medica*, Hu reports that teas, oils and poultices were among the most common treatments used and recorded by both Egyptian and Chinese physicians. I think it is no coincidence that even over great geographical distances and among people of vastly different cultures, ancient physicians used many of the same herbal remedies. I believe that human intuition once played a greater role in people's lives and common sense dictated their treatment modalities.

In contrast, science dominates culture today. If scientific studies cannot quantitatively *prove* that something is right or true, many people do not accept that it is right. Even if common sense says something is right, scientists argue that it is not, because it cannot be proven. I believe it is wrong to abandon the past and traditions simply because modern science currently lacks the tools to irrevocably prove how a food might work as medicine. The traditional methods for using foods as medicines that I outline in this book make sense—and I think you will recognize many of them, which we have adapted to everyday use. You might be surprised to find just how much of herbal medicine culture has found its way into the halls of medicine. The key is to remember that our food and our medicine can be one and the same.

Applications of Herbal Medicine

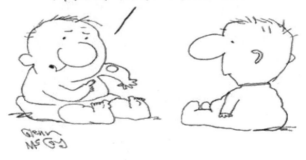

Several methods can be used for administering herbal treatments and modalities. In order to help you understand the basic names of many herbal treatments, I have written a brief description of the most commonly used forms. Although over 15 modalities of treatment exist, many of them are too time-consuming to be practical or too "wacky" (a really scientific term) to recommend. I commonly use five modalities, which I have included in this book.

Some of these treatments can be prepared in just a few minutes and some may take up to an hour. As a home pharmacy beginner, it is important to follow the directions closely when making a remedy. Don't forget, these remedies are time tested. Following the recommendations outlined in this book is similar to following the instructions on an OTC or prescription medication. If you want it to work, you have to use it the right way and for the right purpose. However, just like a cooking recipe, with practice and experience you can modify each remedy to best fit your needs. The main difference between herbal medicine and prescription drug use is that you probably won't die if you make a mistake in the use of an herb. Documented deaths due to herbal medicines are typically very rare, whereas documented deaths due to prescription drug use or overuse number over 26,000 each year, according to the Centers for Disease Control (CDC).

The five modalities for herbal treatments that are the most practical and the least time-consuming are as follows:

- Teas
- Tinctures
- Oils
- Salves and Lip Balms
- Poultices

Teas

The remedies I use most often are medicinal teas. Teas are simple remedies that can alleviate, treat or cure most common illnesses. Teas are simple, effective and generally safe to use every day. However, learning the proper type of tea to make different types of medicine is very important in order to get the right potency or the right treatment for the ailment.

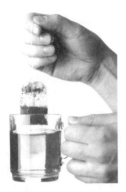

Using a tea bag is a common type of infusion.

There are two common means of making medicinal teas: infusions and decoctions.

Infusions are liquid solutions of plant extracts prepared by pouring boiling liquid over the plant material. Infusions are the most common herbal remedy. Many people use infusions every day without realizing it—tea made with tea bags is an infusion, as is instant coffee. It is not necessary to use water as the liquid when making an infusion. I commonly use apple juice in order to get my children to drink the herbal remedies I make for them.

To make an infusion, simply place the plant material listed in the recipe in a cup or in a strainer over a cup and pour the hot liquid over it. Another way to make an infusion is to add the herb into a pot of hot (not boiling) water and let it sit for up to 10 minutes. Strain the plant material from the pot and drink the liquid. Infusions are great for materials such as leaves, flowers, fresh fruit and other matter in which nutrients can be easily extracted with heat and water.

Jasmine tea, chamomile tea and peppermint tea are common infusions and have great medicinal benefits. Using infusions multiple times a day when no ailment is present, however, is like taking medicine unnecessarily. Over long periods of time, it may be disadvantageous. For example, goldenseal, which contains the alkaloids berberine and hydrastine, should not be taken for more than three weeks in a row because it may unnecessarily stimulate the immune system.

Decoctions are types of herbal teas made from plant material

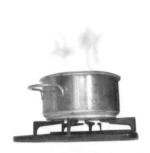

that is woody, rough and tough, such as seeds, stems, bark, dried fruit and roots. The nutrients in these types of materials cannot be extracted effectively through infusion methods but require extended periods of heating. A decoction is prepared by boiling the material in water for 20–30 minutes and then simmering for another 10 minutes or longer. The lid is typically kept on the pot the entire time. This

Decoctions must be boiled for an extended time to extract nutrients.

allows tougher herbs to soften so the water can extract the nutrients contained within. Because decoctions take more time, they are not used as commonly as infusions. But decoctions are just as effective as infusions, if not more so, because seeds, roots, stems and bark contain many beneficial phytochemicals with medicinal properties.

For most decoctions, a standard ratio of material to water is 1:20 by volume (one part material to 20 parts water). This would mean that if you use 1/4 cup of material, you would need to add five cups of water. Follow the recipe as closely as possible the first few times you make it, but just as a seasoned chef may make small changes here and there to a dish, once you are familiar with the recipe you may add or take away according to your own intuition and needs.

Tinctures

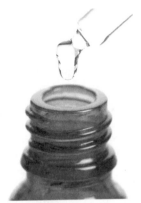

Store tinctures in sterile amber containers to protect from spoilage from bacteria and light.

Tinctures have been produced and used since the beginning of recorded time. They are a great way of turning plants and foods into medicine. Making them requires a bit of time, but there are many reasons to consider taking the time to make a tincture. Among them are portability, excellent shelf life, convenience and efficacy. Having a few homemade tinctures in your medicine cabinet could save a lot of money and time in fewer trips to an allopathic doctor.

Perhaps the best way to describe a tincture is to call it a "pickled" plant. Tinctures are concentrated extracts of medicinal plants that use alcohol, vinegar or glycerin as the means of extraction. Alcohol is the best means of extraction in most cases. However, those who might be sensitive to using alcohol or who will not use it for religious reasons will get some value by using either vinegar or glycerin. During the process of pickling, the alcohol, vinegar or glycerin leaches nutrients from the plant. After days, weeks or even months of soaking the plant in the solution, the liquid extract that results is known as a tincture. Many modern cough remedies, such as Robitussin® and NyQuil®, reportedly originated from tinctures (thus the high alcohol content of these remedies).

Method for making a tincture:

Because of the water contained in plant material, to make an effective tincture you will need to use at least 95 percent (190-proof) alcohol (Everclear®, vodka or brandy is sufficient). If 190-proof alcohols are not available, let the plant material wilt or dry thoroughly before using your alternative alcohol source. Use one part material to two parts liquid, by weight (i.e., one ounce herb to two ounces alcohol).

1. Chop the plant material into dime-sized pieces.
2. Place plant material in a jar with alcohol.
3. Seal the jar with a tight-fitting lid.
4. Let it sit for 10–14 days.
5. After 10 days or longer, strain the liquid into 1 or 2 ounce amber colored glass containers (a cheesecloth or coffee filter works well for straining). Amber or darker bottles are best since some active phytochemicals are sensitive to lights and may be rendered inactive if exposed to light. Squeeze the filter (with the material in it) well to get all of the juice out of the material.
6. Store in a cool, dark place (such as a medicine cabinet) for use as needed.

Tinctures are used very differently from teas. Take small drops throughout the day for illnesses. Because tinctures contain alcohol, vinegar or glycerin, do not overuse them. Keep them out of the reach of children.

Oils

Before we begin to discuss oils, you need to understand the typical terms used to define various types of oils. There is a huge difference between essential oils and herbal oils.

Essential oils are distilled volatile oils of plants. Most essential oils on the market cannot be ingested because of impurities in the distillation process or because of oil-based chemicals such as herbicides and pesticides used in the growing operation of the raw plant material. However, a 100 percent pure essential oil with no impurities may be safely ingested and may be quite effective as a medicinal modality. *Since some essential oils are toxic, use caution when ingesting them. Ingest only therapeutic grade oils and follow all directions on product packaging.*

Making an essential oil requires special equipment and typically cannot be done at home so I will not focus on it in this book. However, many pure essential oils can be purchased readily at your local health food store and online. Of the many companies I have reviewed, there is only one that tests its oils for any impurities. I include this source in the "Suppliers" section on page 151.

Herbal oils are easily made at home and are an important part of creating your own "home pharmacy." Herbal oils can be used as a topical oil or can serve as your base for the production of herbal salves and various massage oils. These oils are great for ear infections, acne, eczema, stiff muscles and many other simple ailments. If you want to make a salve, as explained in the next section, start by making an herbal oil. In order to make an herbal oil, you will need a *fixed oil.*

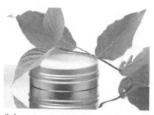

Salves are a convenient application of herbal medicines.

Fixed oils are solvents used to draw out active chemicals in plants. Olive oil is one of the most common fixed solvents. Grapeseed oil, almond oil and apricot kernel oil are other widely used fixed oils. First-press extra virgin olive oil is my fixed oil or solvent of choice, and if I cannot find any, I use grapeseed oil. By combining fixed oils with herbs you can make great massage oils, and then from there, use them to make lotions, lip balms and many other beneficial salves.

Method for making herbal oils:

Use only dried herbs for making an herbal oil. As a general rule, use three ounces of the herb for one pint of fixed oil. There is a lot of leeway with herbal oils, so feel free to experiment with these ratios.

1. Place the herbs in a jar and completely fill the jar with the fixed oil, covering the herbs with at least two inches of oil. Do not allow space for air at the top—purchase jars of the proper size for your batch. Screw the lid on tightly.
2. Leave in a warm, sunny spot such as a windowsill for at least two weeks. The oil will take on the color and taste of whatever herb used.

Salves and Lip Balms

Herbal salves have been used for thousands of years because they are safe and effective. They are an excellent choice for pain relief or for any type of insect bite, burn, itching or skin irritation.

Most people use commercial herbal salves and oils every day, but there are many other effective medicinal oils and salves that are less known. This is largely due to the current label laws, which restrict information on the label. The structure/function claim laws are a good example. Under the DSHEA (Dietary Supplement Health and Education Act), a food or food supplement cannot make any claim outside of the normal function or structure of the body. In other words, an herbal immunity boosting formula cannot say it helps boost the immune system. It must say it "supports the normal function of the immune system." Or a joint pain herbal formula cannot claim it alleviates pain. It must say something like "supports the normal function of healthy joints."

Because salves are so handy (and economical), try taking a Saturday afternoon with your kids to make a year's supply.

Method for making herbal salves:

To make an herbal salve from your herb of choice:

1. Using the prepared herbal oil (see page 40), strain the herb from the oil using cheesecloth or a fine strainer.
2. Place the herbal oil in the upper pan of a double boiler. Add 1/4 cup of beeswax for every cup of the oil. *(Do not use paraffin wax.)*
3. Melt the herbal oil and beeswax together and check the

consistency by dipping the end of a teaspoon into the mixture and allowing the small portion on the spoon to cool. It should feel like a lip salve when cool. If it is too soft, add more beeswax. If it is too firm, add more oil.

4. Prepare containers to pour the salve into while it is still hot and in liquid form. Be sure to label them, listing the ingredients and the date produced. Small one-ounce containers work best for burn creams and lip salves used occasionally, but if you are making a salve for arthritic or joint pain, use a four-ounce or an eight-ounce jar depending on how frequently you will use the salve.

5. Store in a cool, dark place such as a cupboard.

Method for making lip balm:

1. Add one tablespoon of each of the following into a double boiler:

avocado oil   mango butter
coconut oil   shea butter
sweet almond oil   beeswax

(You may substitute any oil or butter you prefer. Other options include olive oil, sesame oil, hemp seed butter, cocoa butter, etc. Oils and butters vary in consistency, so experiment to get the texture and firmness you desire.)

Optional: Add a 1/2 tablespoon of lanolin for a waterproof effect.

2. Melt oils and butters together.

3. After the oils and butters are melted, add one milliliter or 16 drops of an essential oil of your choice.

4. Mix well and pour into containers.

The feeling of making your own salve or lip balm is something everyone should experience. It is easy and a great activity for kids to participate in as well. The pride they will feel as they use their handmade lip balm at school and show it to their friends will not be easily forgotten. Making salves and other skin care items can be a fun family experience.

Poultices

A poultice is a warm, moist mass of powdered or cut herbs that is applied directly to a wound or injury, allowing the medicinal properties of the herbs to be absorbed into the body through the skin. *A poultice is always used externally.* Poultices are beneficial for burns, cuts, swelling and inflammation, rashes, insect and snake bites, fungal infections, acne and many other surface conditions.

Poultices are widely used in allopathic medicine today. Have you ever used a nicotine patch, a menthol pad, a hormone patch or a birth control patch? A medicinal patch was originally derived from a poultice. The skin, as an organ, is able to absorb into the bloodstream many beneficial nutrients that can assist in the healing of injuries or ailments. Only 50 years ago, allopathic medicine taught that the skin could not breathe or absorb. Science finally caught up with herbal medicine, and poultices (or patches) are a trend in pharmaceutical drug delivery systems.

Method for making an herbal poultice:

Option 1

1. Make a strong decoction of herbs of your choice.
2. Let the decoction cool to lukewarm.
3. Soak a cotton cloth in the decoction.
4. Apply the cloth to the affected area.

Option 2

1. Crush or grind fresh herbs, a small amount of water, olive oil or 190-proof alcohol to make a thick paste.
2. Apply the paste to the wound or injury.
3. Cover the pasted wound with a warm cloth or gauze and lightly tape or tie it into place.

Use for minor conditions only. For serious health concerns, visit a healthcare practitioner immediately.

Becoming a "Home Pharmacist"

Teas, tinctures, oils, salves and poultices are the most common methods of using foods and herbs as medicine. Other methods are found in references such as *School of Natural Healing* by Dr. John R. Christopher (one of my personal favorites) or *The Healing Power of Herbs* by Dr. Michael T. Murray. However, many of the methods outlined in these books are quite uncomfortable (such as herbal suppositories) and require some training and skill to use.

I don't expect anyone to simply read this book and become an expert on the use of herbs overnight. Making herbal remedies is a lot like cooking. Truly, anyone can do it, but it takes skill, practice and some patience to become adept at it. Soon you will be improvising and adding to the recipes in this book as you begin to experiment with combinations of different herbs. Test new creations on yourself and experiment to learn which herbs work for certain ailments and which may not. Soon you will have your own collection of do-it-yourself remedies.

The more you experiment, the more you will see that herbal remedies are effective and easy to make. You will also find that if you misuse an herbal remedy, the consequences are typically not dire. In the worst case scenario, you may end up having to take a few more trips to the bathroom if you accidentally combine the wrong herbs for the wrong problem. Over time, using herbs as medicine can save you time, frustration and money. Your new knowledge will help you take charge of your life and give you confidence in your role as the parent (and therefore the primary caregiver) of your family. See pages 69–111 for ideas of which herbs are most effective for which conditions.

Tools for Your Home Pharmacy

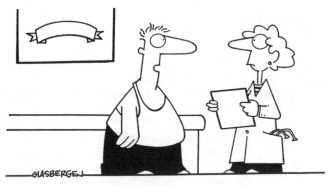

"I must be eating right. I'm narrow at the top and wide at the bottom, just like the food pyramid."

In order to make herbal recipes, you will need some "tools of the trade." Don't worry; you may already have most of the items you will need to begin. Most ingredients aren't expensive and are easily found in any kitchen store. To make things simple, I have recommended some mail-order suppliers who carry these tools in the "Suppliers" section in Appendix B on page 151. You will also need access to the herbs listed in the recipes you want to use. Many of the herbs can be found in the produce section of a grocery store, and you may even be able to find a few in your backyard. Try growing the rest in your own herbal garden (see Appendix A on page 141 for information on growing your own herbs) or finding a local herb shop or health food store that sells bulk herbs. For items you can't grow yourself or find locally, a list in Appendix B on page 151 contains suppliers for herbs, bottles and various other products you may need.

Good Tools

- Wooden or stainless steel spoons
- Stainless steel cookware (mixing bowl, 1 or 2 quart pot, double boiler)
- Cheesecloth, coffee filters or other types of strainers

- Food scale with an ounce/gram converter
- Glass cups for teas; glass jars and small glass bottles for salves, ointments and tinctures (**no plastic**)

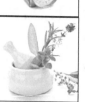

- A mortar and pestle to grind herbs into powder (optional)
- Some time and patience

Do not spend hundreds of dollars on elaborate items. Simple tools are often the easiest to use and may be purchased at most kitchen supply stores.

Common Medicinal Herbs

Below is a list of herbs and other food items you should never be without. You may be surprised to learn how many you may already have. It is amazing what knowledge can do for you. Once you learn that the foods you use every day can also be made into medicines, you may never view food the same way again. These simple herbs, when combined in different ways, can treat most ailments from the common cold or flu to fungal or viral infections. Here is the list of herbs, spices and foods your kitchen should always include.

- fresh garlic or garlic bulbs
- oregano or oregano oil
- ginger root
- cayenne pepper
- dandelion roots
- lemongrass
- echinacea roots (the common coneflower, which looks lovely in a garden)
- sage (like the common sagebrush or other varieties)
- peppermint
- aloe vera (make sure you own an aloe vera plant and not another variety of aloe)
- rose hips
- cinnamon
- raw honey
- lemons or limes

Herbs with antibiotic properties:

- echinacea
- oregano
- garlic
- lemongrass

Herbs with antifungal properties:

- ginger
- garlic
- sage
- rosemary

Herbs that work as antivirals:

- garlic
- lemongrass
- sage

Herbs that function as diuretics:

- dandelion
- ginger
- lemongrass
- aloe vera gel

Herbs that work as relaxants:

- peppermint
- ginger
- chamomile

If you have the space to grow other herbs, dozens more would be beneficial, but the previously-mentioned herbs are the prime healers. Many people are surprised to learn how common these herbs are. Many are foods we use every day. Don't forget, as Hippocrates noted long ago, our food is our medicine!

Essential Home Pharmacy Herbs

(See Appendix A on page 141 for instructions on growing these herbs)

Aloe Vera

(*Aloe vera* or *Aloe barbadensis*)
Aloe vera is a plant with thick green leaves that grows throughout Africa. It is cultivated in Japan for its curative properties.

Active Phytochemicals

Aloe vera contains a number of biologically-active compounds that have been found to increase collagen production, reduce inflammation and assist in healing by increasing levels of fibrinogen (a protein produced by the liver that helps blood clots to form).

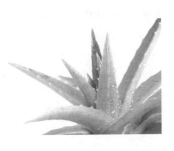

History and Traditional Use
Humans have valued aloe vera for thousands of years. Images of aloe vera are found in carvings in Egyptian temples from the fourth

millennium BC, and the *Egyptian Book of Remedies* from 1500 BC suggests aloe vera for treating infections and skin problems. Aloe vera is used in traditional Chinese medicine and Ayurvedic medicine. It is used in Arabic medicine for treating fevers.

Aloe vera became popular in the United States in the 1930s as a remedy for treating X-ray burns. It is still widely used in traditional herbal remedies across the globe for its soothing properties. Aloe vera gel, contained inside the leaves of the plant, is commonly used topically to support treatment of minor burns, including sunburn. The gel has also been used to soothe stings, cuts and skin irritation. Apply a thin layer of aloe vera gel to the affected area. Aloe vera gel has moisturizing properties and is a common ingredient in lotions. Aloe vera leaf, on the other hand, has been used in the United States as a laxative since the 1800s. Aloe vera leaves (not the gel) contain *aloin*, a powerful laxative.

Recent Scientific Studies

Aloe vera gel is often recommended as a liquid supplement to provide support for inflammatory bowel diseases such as Crohn's disease and ulcerative colitis. A study published in *Alimentary Pharmacology & Therapeutics* found that aloe vera gel had an anti-inflammatory action, supporting this use.

Research also supports the topical use of aloe vera gel to treat skin disorders. A 2008 study in *Journal of Drugs in Dermatology* reported that aloe vera gel is beneficial in treating psoriasis and other skin disorders.

Note: Taken orally, aloe vera leaf can cause diarrhea and cramps. For skin disorders, use the gel topically. When taking the leaf as a laxative, use with caution.

Cayenne Pepper

(*Capsicum frutescens* or *Capsicum annuum*)

Cayenne pepper is a hot chili pepper, originally grown in tropical regions of the Western hemisphere. The pepper is made by grinding the dried fruit to powder. The pungency of cayenne can vary—typically, the more tropical the climate, the more pungent (or "hot") the spice, but hot peppers can grow anywhere.

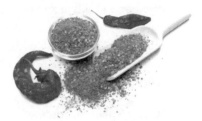

Active Phytochemicals

Like most hot peppers, cayenne peppers contain capsaicin, a pungent natural chemical found in many topical creams for arthritis pain. Cayenne pepper is also high in vitamin A and contains vitamin B_6, vitamin C, vitamin E, riboflavin, potassium and manganese.

History and Traditional Use

Cayenne was first described by a physician who traveled to the Caribbean with Christopher Columbus (1451–1506) in the 15th century. The explorers brought cayenne peppers back to Europe, and Europeans began substituting cayenne pepper for black pepper, which was very expensive. Cayenne peppers now grow throughout the world and are used both as a spice for cooking and for their healing properties.

If you've ever felt your face flush and your nose start to drip while eating spicy foods, you've experienced some of the most fundamental uses of cayenne pepper. Cayenne pepper increases circulation and blood flow to the skin and helps break down mucus buildup. Therefore, it is often used to relieve symptoms of colds and sinus infections. Cayenne pepper also stimulates digestion and aids in the absorption of nutrients, so it is effective for constipation and gas and may also increase the efficacy of other herbal remedies. Cayenne can be taken orally as a dietary supplement or used as an ingredient in poultices to ease muscles aches and pain.

Recent Scientific Studies

A 2009 study published in *Acta Oto-Laryngologica* reported that cayenne can be beneficial for nonallergic rhinitis (chronic congestion, sneezing and drippy nose, similar to hay fever but with no apparent cause). The study found that a nasal spray containing cayenne (capsicum) administered three times a day reduced symptoms in these patients.

Taken orally, cayenne may also have the potential to reduce symptoms in people suffering from chronic indigestion. In a study published in *Alimentary Pharmacology and Therapeutics* in 2002, patients received 2.5 grams of cayenne powder a day before meals. The patients reported experiencing fewer symptoms of indigestion.

Cayenne is also often an ingredient in many topical preparations for pain. In 2007, researchers studied the efficacy of various herbal treatments for lower back pain. The researchers reported in the journal *Spine* that applying an ointment containing *C. frutescens* helped reduce pain in the subjects of the study.

Cinnamon

(*Cinnamomum* spp.)

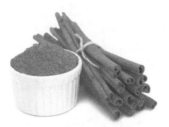

Cinnamon is a common spice that comes from the bark of a tree native to Southeast Asia.

Active Phytochemicals

Cinnamon contains several phytochemicals. Among the most active compounds are cinnamtannin B_1, which helps combat free radicals; eugenol, an essential oil with antiseptic properties often used in flavorings and perfumes; and cinnamic aldehyde, an organic compound that can help prevent unwanted clumping of blood platelets. Cinnamon is also high in manganese, a mineral essential to healthy nerves and proper blood sugar regulation.

History and Traditional Use

Most people ingest quite a bit of cinnamon during a lifetime. But many people don't know that in addition to spicing up holiday recipes and adding a unique flavor to drinks and desserts, cinnamon has also been used as an herbal remedy for centuries. Cinnamon was imported from China to Egypt around 2000 BC, and subsequently the use of the spice spread throughout Europe. In medieval times, cinnamon was used as a preservative.

Cinnamon has many medicinal uses in addition to its value as a spice. It has been used to increase circulation and help with gastrointestinal problems. Cinnamon was also valued historically as an antibacterial agent.

Recent Scientific Studies

A recent study, published in the *Journal of Agriculture and Food Chemistry* in 2005, reported that cinnamon may also be effective as an antibiotic. Cinnamon has been studied for use as an antifungal. A 2008 study published in the *Canadian Journal of Microbiology* reported that cinnamon, as an essential oil, was a potent treatment for *Candida albicans*, a common intestinal yeast that causes yeast infections.

Another recent clinical study published in 2003 in *Diabetes Care* found that cinnamon can be a good treatment for type 2 diabetes. In this study, a daily dose of cinnamon reduced not only blood sugar levels, but also cholesterol levels in people with type 2 diabetes. Don't attempt to treat type 2 diabetes without consulting a physician, but if you are diagnosed with it, you may consider increasing your cinnamon intake under the direction of a healthcare practitioner.

Dandelion

(*Taraxacum officinale*)
Dandelion root comes from a plant related to chicory that grows commonly throughout the United States. It is commonly thought to be a weed.

Active Phytochemicals

Dandelion contains phytochemicals such as taraxacin, which aids digestion; inulin, a prebiotic fiber that increases calcium absorption; and phenolic acids. Minerals found in dandelion root include potassium and calcium. Dandelion root is also an excellent source of vitamin A.

History and Traditional Use

Dandelion roots were used by Native Americans in herbal medicinal practices as well as in traditional Arabic medicine. Dandelion root is commonly used for kidney, liver and spleen problems as a tonic and blood purifier that helps the body eliminate toxins. It is a powerful diuretic. In Europe, dandelion roots are used for gastrointestinal problems, as they increase the liver's production of bile, which is vital to proper digestion. The leaves can also be used as food and are found in spring mix salads. They have also been used to treat a wide variety of conditions, from acne to night blindness.

Note: The National Center for Complementary and Alternative Medicine warns not to use dandelion if you have an infected or inflamed gallbladder.

Echinacea Root

(*Echinacea* spp.)

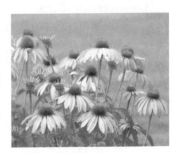

Echinacea, commonly called the purple coneflower, is a flowering plant in the daisy family. It consists of nine species of flowers with medicinal properties.

Active Phytochemicals

The most abundant phytochemical in the *Echinacea* species are polyphenols, a family of natural compounds found in plant foods. Polyphenols found in echinacea root include cichoric acid, which improves immune cell function and quercetin, a natural antihistamine.

History and Traditional Use

Echinacea roots were used historically by Native Americans in the Great Plains region. Early European settlers to the region adopted the use of echinacea to treat dizziness and purify the blood. Over the past decades, echinacea has increased in popularity as a way to boost the immune system, particularly against colds and flu during season changes.

Recent Scientific Studies

Several recent studies report that echinacea may be useful in preventing and fighting upper respiratory tract infections. A 2007 study published in *Lancet Infectious Diseases* reported that echinacea supplements may have the potential to support common cold treatments. The study reported that those taking echinacea were less likely to contract colds, and when they did get colds, the duration was shorter.

Note: Avoid echinacea if you are allergic to plants in the daisy family, including ragweed.

Garlic

(*Allium sativum*)
Garlic is an edible bulb from the lily family that is commonly used in both food and medicine.

Active Phytochemicals

Garlic contains a potent antibacterial agent known as allicin. Numerous clinical studies, including a 1999 study in *Microbes and Infection* and another published in 2009 in the *British Journal of Biomedical Science*, show allicin to be an effective bacterial fighter.

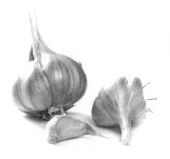

History and Traditional Use

Even though many people associate garlic with bad breath more readily than with medicine, this herb has been used as both an antibiotic and an antifungal for millennia. Ancient Greek physicians used garlic, and garlic is important in traditional Chinese medicine. Garlic was used as an antimicrobial to treat wounds and infections and prevent gangrene in both World Wars. As one of the longest-standing and most basic herbal remedies, fresh garlic has historically been used for a wide variety of conditions, from coughing to gangrene and from infections to intestinal worms.

Recent Scientific Studies

Numerous studies substantiate the use of garlic to lower blood pressure and cholesterol and prevent heart disease. In 2008, a study published in *The Annals of Pharmacotherapy* reported that garlic lowered blood pressure in people with high blood pressure. A 2010 study published in *Lipids in Health and Disease* reported that garlic powder tablets significantly decreased cardiovascular risk in patients, particularly in men.

Note: Garlic can thin the blood, so avoid taking garlic supplements within a few weeks before or after surgery.

Ginger

(*Zingiber officinale*)

Ginger is a plant with green-purple flowers. The root (called a rhizome) is commonly used in both medicine and cooking.

Active Phytochemicals

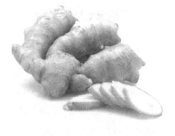

Ginger contains an active phytochemical called zingerone, which is effective against *Escherichia coli* (commonly known as *E. coli*). Additionally, ginger contains shogaol and gingerol, phytochemicals that help reduce fevers and suppress coughing. Shogaol and gingerol compose one to three percent of the weight of fresh ginger and give the herb its distinctive smell and spicy taste. Ginger also contains compounds called sesquiterpenes, which are effective against the cold virus.

History and Traditional Use

Ginger has been used for thousands of years in traditional medicine in many Asian countries, including China, Japan and India. This herb has many traditional uses—including as a support for stomach aches and diarrhea. Ginger is also used for nausea from motion sickness or pregnancy. Ginger is used to induce fever to kill bacteria. Ginger has antifungal properties and is also commonly used as a diuretic and a muscle relaxant.

Recent Scientific Studies

Clinical studies, including a study published in 1998 in *Archives of Family Medicine*, found that the phytochemical gingerol increases the body's ability to move food through the gastrointestinal tract and has painkilling, sedative, fever-reducing and antibacterial properties.

Other recent studies have looked at ginger's anti-nausea properties. In 2006, a study published in *Pharmacology* reported that ginger reduced nausea associated with morning sickness in pregnant women. Also in 2006, a study published in the *Journal of the Medical Association of Thailand* reported that patients who took ginger supplements before surgery experienced less post-surgery nausea than people who did not take ginger.

Lemongrass

(*Cymbopogon citratus*)

Lemongrass is a tall grass native to Asia. Freshly cut and partially dried leaves are used in medicine as well as cooking.

Active Phytochemicals

Organic chemicals including geraniol, which has been shown to slow cancer growth, and citronellol, which has antibacterial and anti-inflammatory properties, are found in lemongrass. Citronellol is the best known of these chemicals.

In animal studies, citronellol was found to lower blood pressure. Lemongrass also contains citral, a compound that is responsible for its lemony scent and shows antioxidant activity in animal studies.

History and Traditional Use

Lemongrass is also known as lemon verbena and fever grass. In the United States, lemongrass is often referred to as citronella (*Cymbopogon nardus* and *Cymbopogon winterianus*), a popular ingredient in scent-based mosquito repellents. Lemongrass is one of the most widely used plants in South American folk medicine, and it is commonly used in Asian cooking. Historically it was used as a digestive aid, since it helps remove toxins from organs such as the liver, bladder, pancreas and kidneys and stimulates blood circulation. It is also effective as an antibiotic and diuretic. Plus, it adds a fresh, lemony aroma to your home that repels insects!

Oregano

(*Origanum vulgare*)

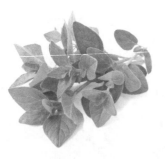

Oregano is an herb in the mint family with purple flowers. It is typically dried and used as a spice.

Active Phytochemicals

Phenolic acids (plant compounds with beneficial properties) compose 71 percent of oregano. Such phenolic acids, including rosmarinic acid, protocatechuic acid and caffeic acid, have antioxidant properties. Oregano also contains several flavonoids (naturally-occurring chemical compounds), including carvacrol, thymol, limonene, pinene, ocimene and caryophyllene. Some flavonoids in oregano, such as thymol, have antimicrobial activity. Thymol is a powerful antiseptic agent used in some OTC treatments for acne, and mouth-washes. Oregano is an excellent antiseptic when used topically.

History and Traditional Use

Oregano has long been used in Mexican and Italian food as a spice and flavoring agent and as an ingredient in perfumes and scented soaps. This spice also has a long history of use in natural medicine. It has been used as an antibiotic, antimicrobial, antiseptic, antioxidant and antihistamine. In Morocco, oregano is used in traditional medicine for gastrointestinal disorders. Egyptians use it for food preservation, and oregano is used in Greece to treat various viral disorders. An infusion made with oregano is often used for an upset stomach and indigestion, as well as coughs and respiratory ailments.

Recent Scientific Studies

A study published in the *Journal of International Medical Research* in 2008 reported that a 25 mL dose of liquid oregano extract taken daily over three months increased HDL ("good" cholesterol) and reduced LDL ("bad" cholesterol) in subjects of the study.

A 2007 study published in the *Pakistan Journal of Botany* found that oregano was effective in fighting gram negative bacilli, a class of pathogenic bacteria that frequently cause infections including intestinal inflammation, meningitis and pneumonia. Since these studies are preliminary and it is unclear how effective oregano could be against such bacteria, see a healthcare practitioner if you suspect you are infected.

Note: Avoid large amounts oregano (as tea or decoction) if you are pregnant, as it can induce miscarriage.

Peppermint

(*Mentha* × *piperita*)

Active Phytochemicals

Peppermint is a source of menthol, an organic compound found in many antiseptic and local anesthetic preparations. Menthol can reduce throat and mouth irritation and relieve minor muscle aches and pains.

History and Traditional Use

Peppermint has been used both as food and as a natural remedy for thousands of years. Peppermint, a cross between watermint and spearmint, was introduced in medical literature in the 17th century, but records from ancient Greece, Egypt and Rome show that these ancient cultures used relatives of peppermint in herbal medicine. Chewing on a peppermint leaf can calm an upset stomach and relieve a headache, not to mention improve breath. Peppermint also has a calming, soothing effect on the nerves and is a great stress reliever. Peppermint is commonly used as a flavoring in chewing gum, toothpaste and mouthwash and is found in some cough and cold remedies.

Recent Scientific Studies

In 2000, a study published in *Alimentary Pharmacology and Therapeutics* found that peppermint reduced heartburn symptoms and pain. Subjects of the study were given a combination of peppermint oil (90 mg) and caraway oil (50 mg).

Peppermint may also help with a variety of digestive disorders by improving gastric emptying, meaning that the stomach content passes into the intestines more quickly. A 2008 study published in *BMJ* reported that peppermint oil helped relieve symptoms related to irritable bowel syndrome (IBS).

Rose Hips

(*Rosa* spp.)

Rose hips are the bulbous growths that appear on many types of rose bushes after the rose petals have withered away.

Active Phytochemicals

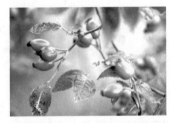

Rose hips are extremely high in vitamin C if harvested at maturity, and are therefore very useful in fighting infection. Since rose hips are high in vitamins A, C and E, they have antioxidant properties. Rose hips also contain fatty acids and many bioflavonoids such as lycopene, an antioxidant. Betulin, another compound found in rose hips, helped lower cholesterol in animal studies.

History and Traditional Use

Rose hips have been an important food source for native tribes anywhere roses grow. Rose hips were a popular remedy for chest ailments during the Middle Ages (1000–1300 AD). Historically rose hips have also been quite effective in treating scurvy and all infections. Other uses include reducing stress, treating dizziness and headaches and strengthening the heart.

Recent Scientific Studies

A large body of research supports the use of rose hips to strengthen immune function. One early study, published in *Mechanisms of Ageing and Development*, reported that isolated constituents of rose hips increased the activity of the immune system's natural killer cells.

Recent scientific research shows that rose hips have anti-inflammatory properties. A 2005 study published in the *Scandinavian Journal of Rheumatology* reported that a powder made from seeds and shells of rose hips reduced hip and knee osteoarthritis. A subsequent study, published in *Phytotherapy Research* in 2008 found that a powder made from rose hip and seed powder reduced symptoms of long-term pain for patients suffering from osteoarthritis.

Sage

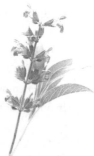

(*Salvia officinalis*)
Sage is a small, evergreen plant native to the Mediterranean. It has violet flowers.

Active Phytochemicals

Powerful antiseptics cineole and borneol are the main phytochemical oils in sage. There are dozens of other phytochemicals in sage including niacin, oleic acid and caffeine.

History and Traditional Use

Sage is perhaps one of the oldest documented herbs in European history—Roman emperor Charlemagne (742–814 AD) suggested cultivation of sage for its medicinal properties in the eighth century AD. Traditionally, sage has been used to decrease sweating in people suffering from tuberculosis. It has been used as an antifungal and an antiviral.

Recent Scientific Studies

Sage has traditionally been used to improve cognitive performance in humans. In 2003, a study published in *Pharmacology, Biochemistry and Behavior* reported that a single 50 microliter dose of sage improved short term memory in healthy, young adult volunteers. Also in 2003, in a double-blind, randomized and placebo-controlled trial, published in the *Journal of Clinical Pharmacy and Therapeutics*, researchers found sage to be effective in the management of mild to moderate Alzheimer's disease.

In 2006, a study published in the *European Journal of Medical Research* found that a throat spray containing sage helped soothe sore throats. The spray was a 140 microliter dose of a 15 percent sage solution.

Note: Nursing mothers should avoid sage, as it decreases milk supply.

Your Home Pharmacy

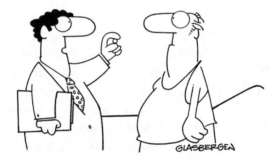

"To prevent a heart attack, take one aspirin every day.
Take it out for a jog, then take it to the gym,
then take it for a bike ride..."

This chapter contains a list of treatments and remedies for various common ailments, alphabetically by ailment. I include recipes for infusions, decoctions, salves and poultices in addition to diet and supplement recommendations. Some of these recipes came from my mother and some came from my father's mother. Some came from watching local healers work in various parts of the world, and others came from my teachers. Among those from whom I have learned directly are David Christopher, son of the prominent doctor of herbal medicine John R. Christopher; the late Dr. Bernard Jensen, father of modern iridology (a technique that uses characteristics of the iris as a way to determine health); David Hoffman, Master Herbalist; Dr. Masazumi Yoshihara, my Japanese pharmacognosy professor and Dr. Yi-Zhun Zhu, dean of pharmacology at Fudan University in Shanghai, China.

As you look for specific ailments in this chapter, please understand that there are hundreds of other ailments I could have included, but this book focuses on remedies for the most common and easily treatable conditions. If you have an ailment for which you cannot find a solution, refer to the "References" on page 153 of this book, where I have included several helpful books. Additionally, my personal e-mail address is included in Appendix B on page 151.

If you have any difficulty making the treatments, I have formulated several of them into supplements that are sold by NutraNomics®, the company I founded. To order any of the supplements from NutraNomics®, refer to the information in the suppliers list at the end of this book, or visit www.nutra-nomics.com.

Again, our society seems to demand instant gratification. Though I have formulated many dietary supplement products for many companies, I always recommend turning first to proper diet and traditional herbal remedies rather than depending on supplements for a quick fix. I view supplements as a crutch. You need a crutch if you have a broken leg. In this case, the broken leg is our unwillingness to change our lifestyles, and the crutch is the dietary supplement. Use the crutch until your broken lifestyle is healed, but make sure you aren't using it to try to avoid having to change your lifestyle. I sometimes use supplements myself, because I don't *always* live and eat as I know I should. Someday I will, but in the meantime I have my crutches.

All of the supplements in the following sections are from NutraNomics® unless noted. See page 110–111 for ingredients in the following formulations.

Acne

Internal

Make an infusion of:

> 2 oz. red clover blossoms
> 1 oz. echinacea root
> 1 oz. nettles root
> 1 oz. burdock root
> 1 oz. dandelion root
> 1/2 oz. licorice root

Steep for 10 minutes in one quart of water, strain and sweeten with honey to taste. Drink three cups a day.

External

Make a facial mask using:

thyme	a little eucalyptus
raw honey	ground avocado skins
carrot pulp	

Apply in the evening before bed for 30 minutes. Rinse mask with warm water. Continue for about one week to see results. Do not worry about quantities of ingredients. Make enough to cover the surface of your face. You will learn the proper quantities as you experiment.

Recommended eating:

Stay away from chemical preservatives and eat lots of green vegetables. Alpha and beta carotenoids (found in yellow and orange foods like apricots, peaches, carrots and sweet potatoes) are also beneficial. Avoid hormone-altering foods such as coffee and chocolate and drink plenty of pure water.

Anemia

Make a decoction of:

1 oz. alfalfa leaves	1/2 oz. pine needles
1 oz. parsley leaves	1/2 oz. dulse
1 oz. dandelion leaves	1/2 oz. burdock root
1 oz. watercress leaves	1 cup unsulfured black-
1/2 oz. yellow dock root	strap molasses

In one quart of apple juice or water, simmer ingredients except molasses for 20 minutes. Let cool and strain. Return liquid to pot, add molasses and simmer for 10 minutes. Place in refrigerator and let cool. Take one tablespoon three times a day.

Note: Avoid pine needles (as a tea or decoction) if you are pregnant, as they can induce miscarriage.

Recommended eating:

Eat plenty of whole-grain foods like whole-grain breads and pastas and dark leafy vegetables like broccoli, mustard greens and collard greens. Eating "red meat" in moderation is also important for anemia but may be harder to digest, so I recommend organic or wild harvested fish. Wild salmon, sardines and fish with darker meat are highest in nutrient content.

Arthritis (Osteo)

The late Dr. Bernard Jensen, who was able to heal himself of many degenerative joint ailments, taught me this wonderful recipe.

Make a soup consisting of:

> veal joint (use a clean, fresh, uncut veal joint
>   washed in cold water)
> potato skins peeled from 2 large potatoes
> 3 stalks of celery
> 1 small onion, chopped
> carrot peelings from 3 large carrots
> 1 handful of parsley leaves

Boil the veal joints for about 30 minutes in about two quarts of water, then add the remaining ingredients and boil for another 30 minutes. Strain off liquid and discard the solid ingredients. Drink two cups of this broth twice a day.

Topically (for pain)
Make a liniment of:

> 1 pint rubbing alcohol
> 1/2 oz. oil of eucalyptus (herbal oil)
> 1/2 oz. oil of wintergreen (herbal oil)

Recommended eating:

Increase the amount of foods containing sodium (*not* salt, which is sodium chloride) and sulfur in your diet. These include apricots, peaches, celery, collard greens, almonds, kelp, goat's milk, dulse, parsley, turnips, Swiss chard, rhubarb stems (*not* the leaves, which are toxic), spring lettuce (young lettuce of any variety), cabbage and real cheeses (meaning those containing enzymes).

Recommended supplements:

Mobility and Flexibility Complex

Athlete's Foot (ringworm, and other topical bacterial and fungal infections)

Make a salve using equal parts (exact amounts will vary depending on the surface area of the infection) of the following:

> oregano
> rosemary
> garlic
> black walnut hulls (the green skin around the walnut)

Apply on infected area at least three times daily.

Recommended eating:

Avoid sweet foods and processed carbohydrates. Eat plenty of green leafy foods like arugula, Swiss chard and kale. Drink lots of water and change your socks and footwear twice daily.

Recommended supplements:

Chaparral capsules* (500 mg daily until the problem is gone)
   Note: Due to potential for liver damage, the FDA cautions against the internal use of chaparral.

*Available from various branded labels at health food stores and online.

Bleeding (external)

Cayenne is the best clotting agent in the natural world. Place powdered cayenne directly onto a wound and bleeding will stop immediately. When an artery has been severed, place cayenne directly over the opening, apply pressure and immediately seek a physician. Don't worry; cayenne only burns in the mouth, anus and eyes but will not burn on an open wound.

After the wound has healed, drink an alfalfa infusion and take flaxseed oil for at least two weeks. This will help restore your iron and platelet levels back to normal.

Recommended eating:

While healing, increase the amount of foods containing iron and sodium (*not* salt) in your diet. These include cherries, spinach, alfalfa, collard greens, almonds, kelp, goat's milk, dulse, parsley, turnips, Swiss chard, rhubarb, spring lettuce and raw (unpasteurized) enzyme-rich dairy products.

Blood Pressure (high)

Make a tincture of the following:

> 3 oz. hawthorn berries
> 1 oz. *Panax ginseng* root
> 1 oz. comfrey root
> 1 oz. mistletoe leaf
> 1 oz. valerian root

Take about 20 drops of this tincture throughout the day.

Note: Due to its pyrrolizidine alkaloid content, people with liver problems should avoid taking comfrey internally.

Recommended eating and lifestyle:

For both high and low blood pressure, I recommend eating a diet high in vegetables and grains. Absolutely avoid all vegetable oils when cooking. Heated polyunsaturated fats and trans-fatty acids—*not saturated fats*—are major contributors to heart disease. Include beneficial fatty acids in your diet and avoid trans-fatty acids, which are found in many fried and processed foods. Check labels for "partially hydrogenated" vegetable oil, an indicator of trans fats. For grains, add rye and barley to your diet. Include foods high in natural potassium and natural sodium (*not* salt) such as apples, beets and greens, black olives, carrots, kale, kelp, lentils, parsley, raisins, sesame seeds, sunflower seeds and Swiss chard.

Other factors can also help manage high blood pressure. Take a hot shower and then turn the water to cold for about five minutes before you finish. Cold water therapy can help constrict blood vessels and stabilize blood pressure. Avoid stress or learn techniques for remaining relaxed under pressure. Balance in life is important.

Recommended supplements:

Red Yeast Rice*
PhytoNutrient
Lipid Systemic Enzyme
All Omega Fat Complex

*Available from various branded labels at health food stores and online.

Blood Pressure (low)

While a less serious medical concern than high blood pressure, low blood pressure can lead to dizziness, light headedness and fatigue. Juices from carrots, beets or celery can help combat such effects because they are all very stimulating. Drink such juices in the morning or whenever you feel tired. Another stimulating drink that may be helpful is "Brigham tea." This tea is made by infusing 1 oz. of dried stems of ephedra (*Ephedra viridis*) in approximately 8 oz. of water. Drink one cup per day.

Increase your water intake to combat dehydration as well as increase blood volume, which can increase blood pressure. Combat dizziness by changing body positions slowly (especially when moving from sitting to standing). Low blood pressure can also cause blood to pool in lower extremities. Compression stockings can help combat this problem.

Burns (first degree)

Immediately after a burn occurs, apply cool water and a sliced aloe vera leaf to stop the burning sensation.

Make a salve of:
> 2 parts comfrey leaves
> 1 part calendula (marigold) flowers

Apply this salve regularly until burning sensation is gone.

Use this approach for mild burns only. For burns with blisters, burns larger than three inches in size, or burns on the hands, face or feet, *seek immediate care from a healthcare practitioner.*

Cancer

The following section contains my thoughts on the treatment of cancer, including some of the research I have reviewed regarding various herbs and their uses against cancer. I have summarized several studies and encourage you to become familiar with the following pages. Through several years of study, I have concluded that natural ATP (adenosine triphosphate) inhibitors combined with Dr. William Kelley's (1925–2005) enzyme therapy are some of the best available methods to support fighting most types of cancer.

Adenosine triphosphate is the energy that cells produce and it is necessary for cellular reproduction. A shortage of ATP will not affect normal slower growing cells but for cancer cells that grow rapidly, a lack of ATP is deadly.

Kelley theorized that a deficiency of pancreatic enzymes (protein molecules that help the body digest food, particularly proteins) may contribute to cancer. Kelley's enzyme therapy protocol combines nutrition, detoxification and supplementation with pancreatic enzymes to boost the body's ability to digest protein and fight cancer. You can find out more about Dr. Kelley's enzyme protocol and his controversial career via the Internet.

Perhaps the best researched ATP inhibitors found naturally are those found in powerful phytochemicals called *annonaceous acetogenins* from the durian fruit (also known as "stinky fruit"), common in Southeast Asia. Acetogenins block or inhibit ATP synthesis in both normal and multidrug resistant cancer cells. Without adequate amounts of ATP, cellular division cannot occur.

To help my clients understand a cell's consumption of ATP,

I compare their cells to automobiles. High-efficiency or hybrid cars can operate for long distances on a small or limited supply of fuel, while SUVs and large trucks have limited range on a similar amount fuel. Likewise normal, healthy cells can operate quite efficiently on a small supply of ATP for a period of months, but cancer cells typically consume 50 to 5,000 times more ATP than normal cells do and will eventually "run out of gas." If rapid cellular division cannot occur, cancer cell growth cannot take place. Cancer cells will eventually die out or be destroyed by the immune system.

Purdue University professor Dr. Jerry McLaughlin stated best how the chemical process of ATP inhibition occurs. McLaughlin wrote:

> "During chemiosmosis in eukaryotes, H+ ions are pumped across an organelle membrane into a confined space [bounded by membranes] that contains numerous hydrogen ions. The energy for the pumping comes from the coupled oxidation-reduction reactions in the electron transport chain. Electrons are passed from one membrane-bound enzyme to another, losing some energy with each transfer (as per the Second Law of Thermodynamics). This "lost" energy allows for the pumping of hydrogen ions against the concentration gradient [there are fewer hydrogen ions outside the confined space than there are inside the confined space]. The confined hydrogens cannot pass back through the membrane. Their only exit is through the ATP-synthesizing enzyme

that is located in the confining membrane. As the hydrogen passes through the ATP-synthesizing enzyme, energy from the enzyme is used to attach a third phosphate to ADP, converting it to ATP. Acetogenins inhibit the ATP synthase enzyme production."

Other research has shown acetogenins to also inhibit ATP distribution, so it may be possible to use these compounds to not only reduce the production of ATP but limit the distribution as well. *ATP inhibitors should not be used as a preventative modality for cancer.* This is a method only for one who has been diagnosed with a rapidly growing cancer. The benefits of acetogenins to cancer patients who are seeking a viable alternative or complement to traditional chemotherapies in my opinion outweigh any other alternative modality for cancer. I have seen their results personally in my own family as well as dozens of friends and clients.

Any treatment for cancer, including the use of ATP inhibitors, should include a change in diet and lifestyle. I also include my views on a healthy diet for those suffering from cancer.

Herbs that provide nutritive support for cancer

Espinheira Santa (Maytansine)

Espinheira santa (*Maytenus ilicifolia*) is a small, shrubby evergreen tree native to South America. The tree can grow up to 15 feet in height and has leaves and berries that resemble holly. Espinheira santa has a much longer and better documented history of use in urban areas and in South American herbal medicine practices than in tribal areas. This is probably because of the types of illnesses it treats. It is also one of the few tropical South American medicinal plants that has been the subject of multiple clinical studies. These studies were fueled by research suggesting the effectiveness of espinheira santa for ulcers and even cancer, documented beginning as early as the mid-1960s. Research suggests that espinheira santa, as well as a few other species in the *Maytenus* genus, contain antibiotic compounds that showed potent antitumor and antileukemic activities at very low dosages.

Two of these compounds, maytansine and mayteine, were tested in cancer patients in the United States and South America during the 1970s. Although there were some significant regressions in ovarian carcinoma and some lymphomas with maytansine, research was discontinued due to the toxicity at the high dosages used. Research with the compound mayteine revealed little to no toxicity and validated its uses in traditional and folk medicine for various types of skin cancers. Cancer research with this compound is still ongoing in South America. In traditional medicine today, an application of the leaves of espinheira santa are employed as an ointment for treating skin cancer and a decoction is used as a wash for skin cancers.

Graviola or Soursop/Guanábana (Acetogenins)

The graviola tree (*Annona* spp.), native to warm areas of South and North America, is a small tree with dark green leaves. It produces a large, heart-shaped, yellow-green fruit with white flesh. A 1976 plant screening program by the National Cancer Institute showed that graviola leaves and stem were poisonous to cancer cells, and researchers have been following up on these findings ever since. Much of the cancer research on graviola focuses on a novel set of phytochemicals called annonaceous acetogenins. Graviola produces these natural compounds in its leaf, stem, bark and fruit seeds. Three separate research groups have isolated these acetogenin compounds in graviola and found that they have significant antitumorous and anticancerous properties and selective toxicity against various types of cancer cells. (Selective toxicity means that these compounds kill cancer cells without harming healthy cells.) These groups have published eight clinical studies on their findings.

Many of the acetogenins demonstrate selective toxicity to tumor cells at very low dosages—as little as one part per million, the equivalent of four drops of liquid in a 55-gallon barrel. Four studies published in 1998 further specify which phytochemicals and acetogenins demonstrate the strongest anticancerous, antitumorous and antiviral properties.

Thus far, specific acetogenins in graviola have been reported to be selectively toxic to the following types of tumor cells: lung carcinoma cell lines, human breast solid tumor lines, prostate adenocarcinoma, pancreatic carcinoma cell lines, colon adenocarcinoma cell lines, liver cancer cell lines and multidrug-resistant human breast adenocarcinomas. Mode-of-action studies in three separate laboratories determined that these acetogenins may stop enzyme processes that are only found in the membranes of cancerous tumor cells.

Researchers at Purdue University have conducted a great deal of the research on the acetogenins, much of which has been funded by The National Cancer Institute or the National Institute of Health. Thus far, Purdue University or its staff has filed at least nine U.S. or international patents on this work concerning the antitumorous and insecticidal properties and uses of these acetogenins.

Researchers in Japan published an interesting study *in vivo* in March of 2002. (*In vivo* studies are performed inside a living organism, in contrast to *in vitro* studies, which are conducted outside living organisms in a controlled environment such as a test tube.) The researchers were studying various acetogenins found in several species of plants. The researchers inoculated mice with a type of lung cancer cell. One third of the mice received no treatment, one third received the allopathic chemotherapy drug Adriamycin®, and one third received the main graviola acetogenin, annonacin, at a dosage of 10 mg/kg (meaning each mouse received 10 mg of annonacin for every kilogram of weight).

At the end of two weeks, the researchers measured lung tumor sizes in all the mice. Five of the six in the untreated control group were still alive. The Adriamycin® group showed a 54.6 percent reduction of tumor mass over the control group—but half of the animals had died from toxicity. The mice receiving annonacin were all still alive, and the tumors were inhibited by 57.9 percent—slightly better than Adriamycin®, and without toxicity.

Cat's Claw

Cat's claw (*Uncaria tomentosa*) is a large, woody vine with small white or red flowers. It gets its name from its hook-like thorns that grow along the vine and resemble the claws of a cat. Cat's claw is indigenous to the Amazon rainforest and other tropical areas of South and Central America.

A 2001 *in vitro* study showed that cat's claw inhibited the growth of a human breast cancer cell line by 90 percent, while another research group reported that it inhibited the binding of estrogens in human breast cancer cells *in vitro*. In a small *in vitro* trial in 1998, Swedish researchers documented that cat's claw inhibited the growth of lymphoma and leukemia cells.

In observatory trials in the early 1970s, Austrian researcher Klaus Keplinger found that cancer patients who took cat's claw in conjunction with traditional cancer therapies such as chemotherapy and radiation reported fewer side effects to the traditional therapies (such as hair loss, weight loss, nausea, secondary infections and skin problems). Subsequent researchers have shown how these effects might be possible. They have reported that cat's claw may aid in DNA cellular repair and prevent cells from mutating; it also can help *leucopenia,* the loss of white blood cells and damage to the immune system that is a common side effect of many chemotherapy drugs.

Maitake (Beta-Glucans)

Beta-glucans found in the maitake mushroom (*Grifola frondosa*) respond to tumor cells by stimulating the production of cytokines, which are small protein substances within the phagocytic cells (white blood cells vital to fighting infection). Cytokines stimulate the macrophages (white blood cells that help destroy tumors by absorbing waste materials) to inhibit tumor cell replication and kill the tumor.

Because beta-glucan activates macrophages and T-cells (white blood cells that destroy invaders in the body), researchers have used it as an anticancer treatment by itself, or as a non-toxic complement to chemotherapy. In a 1985 study in *Hepatology*, researchers administered beta-glucan intravenously to mice and injected the mice with tumor cells. The researchers found that tumors were less likely to spread to the livers of animals that were treated with beta-glucan compared with control animals. By the end of the 50 day study period, the mice treated with beta-glucan had a 28 percent increase in survival compared to those not treated with beta-glucan.

Although most research on beta-glucan has been done with animals, there have been a number of human studies. In 1975, the *Journal of the National Cancer Institute* reported on the anticancer effects of beta-glucan in nine cancer patients who suffered from skin, breast or lung cancer. Researchers injected beta-glucan directly into the tumors. In all cases, beta-glucan reduced the size of the tumor within five days. This happens because immune cells infiltrate the cancerous area, subsequently destroying the cancer cells.

A number of clinical studies have been conducted in Japan with lentinan, which is derived from the shiitake mushroom. In Japan, lentinan is approved for medicinal use. Japanese scientists treating advanced cancer patients with lentinan by intravenous injection, increased the number and activity of immune natural killer cells and potentially prolonged survival—sometimes in excess of five or more years.

According to researchers at the National Cancer Center in Japan, tumors were completely eliminated in about 80 percent of cancer-induced animals that were fed extracts from maitake, shiitake and reishi mushrooms. Compounds of each of these mushrooms increase the tumor-fighting activity of natural killer cells of the immune system and improve antibody responses, but maitake seems to have the strongest and most consistent effect. Unlike other mushroom extracts, maitake extract shows strong anticancer activity even when administered orally.

Mutamba (Procyanidin B-2)

The mutamba tree (*Guazuma ulmifolia*) has a long history of indigenous use in Mexico, where it is called *guasima* or *guacima*. A phytochemical analysis of mutamba bark shows that it is a rich source of the natural chemical compound procyanidin B-2, and other biological activities have been documented as well. Of particular note, in 1990 a Brazilian research group demonstrated that a crude extract of mutamba was cytotoxic to cancer cells, exhibiting a 97.3 percent inhibition rate. Later independent research showed that procyanidin B-2 also demonstrated anti-tumorous and anticancerous effects (even against melanoma) as well as blood pressure reducing and kidney protective properties.

Suma (Pfaffic Acids)

The suma root (*Pfaffia paniculata*) contains novel phytochemicals including saponins, pfaffic acids, glycosides and nortriterpenes. The specific saponins found in the roots of suma include a group of phytochemicals called pfaffosides that have demonstrated an ability to inhibit cultured tumor cell melanomas (*in vitro*). The pfaffosides and pfaffic acid derivatives in suma were patented as antitumor compounds in several Japanese patents in the mid-1980s. In a study described in one of the patents, researchers reported that an oral dosage of 100 mg/kg (of suma saponins) given to rats was active against abdominal cancer. The other patents and Japanese research report that the pfaffic acids found in suma root had a "strong activity" against melanoma, liver carcinoma and lung carcinoma cells at only four to six micrograms of pfaffic acids.

Recommended Diet Changes

Eliminate all meats. Occasional meats are fine for healthy people, but they can inhibit the healing process in those with cancer. Eating fish occasionally (once or twice a week) may be fine, but eat only raw fish (sushi) or fish that is broiled or baked.

Eat lots of dark green leafy vegetables (about six servings a day) and two citrus fruits daily.

One day each week, drink only fresh juiced liquids like barley greens and sprouts or carrot juice and take nutritional supplements as usual.

Eliminate all "white" food (processed food), such as white bread, white pasta, potatoes, white rice and processed sugars. Use whole grains, brown rice, wheat bread, etc., instead.

Supplement Regime

I helped formulate GenEpic™, which is a blend of South American herbs that have been studied for efficacy against cancer. See www.genepic.com for more information.

When you make the previously-recommended dietary changes and take the herbs recommended on pages 80–87, whether in supplement form such as the GenEpic™ program or in whole food form, your digestive system will use less energy, thus allowing this extra energy to be transferred to your immune system to aid in the healing processes.

Recommended Lifestyle Changes

I would also recommend engaging in a stress-relieving exercise such as concentration exercises, meditation or prayer for 15 minutes each day. Extend the time spent on this by five minutes every week. Also, find a hobby that you love (something that makes you happy) and do it at least once a week. Last, but most important, go to bed early (by 10 p.m.) and wake by 6 a.m. All of these things will not only allow your body to heal but will bring balance to the rest of your life as well.

Coordinating With Your Healthcare Practitioner

In case you desire to use these suggestions in place of or to complement chemotherapy, radiation or surgery, please ask your doctor to monitor your progression with the usual routine of magnetic resonance imaging (MRI), CA marker blood tests, computed tomography (CT) scans and/or biopsies. An MRI or CT scan is an actual photo (like an X-ray) of the tumor or cancer mass. Physicians commonly use an MRI or CT scan at the beginning of treatment to get a good idea of the size of the mass. If your herbal treatment is working, the tumor will begin to shrink in size; thus an MRI or CT scan should be able to monitor this reduction in size.

CA markers are antigen markers for specific cancers. There are several markers a physician may monitor before, during and after your treatment. In general, the higher the marker, the more cancer your body is fighting.

However, CA markers are not always an accurate way to monitor growth or reduction of cancer. While such diagnostic tools are still the best way to monitor the growth or decline of cancer, occasionally during the first month or two of alternative treatments, CA markers may actually increase before they drop. This is not always a sign that the cancer is getting worse; it may simply be a sign that your body is producing more antigens to fight the cancer.

As mentioned previously, always discuss your plans for incorporating alternative medicine with your healthcare practitioner and work together to determine a treatment plan and how to monitor your progress. Doing this will avoid confusion and a potential misdiagnosis of your current condition. Biopsies are common when a potential cancerous growth is discovered and usually not necessary again until after the completion of a treatment program or if a curious growth has been discovered elsewhere.

Cholesterol (high or low)

There are two books that everyone in America can benefit from reading: *Cholesterol and Your Health,* by Dr. Chris Mudd, and *Coronary Heart Disease, the Dietary Sense and Nonsense,* by George V. Mann, MD. In these books you will find proof of the great American rip-off regarding a common diet/heart hypothesis. Most Americans believe that plant oils are good for us and animal fats are bad, because of how such fats contribute to cholesterol. But most of our cholesterol levels have to do with genetics.

The raw fact is that when you have an imbalance in your HDL-to-LDL ratios, cholesterol—a steroid alcohol, not a fat—contributes to the buildup of plaque in the blood, clogging the arteries and potentially leading to a stroke. Cholesterol is not the only reason for strokes and clogged arteries but is a contributing factor. The proper ratio of HDL to LDL is that HDL should equal 20 percent of your total cholesterol levels plus or minus 3 percent (i.e., a total cholesterol count of 300 is fine if your HDL is 60 and your LDL is 240).

If you want your blood cholesterol ratios to balance out, try the following:

1. Remove all trans-fatty acids from your diet (i.e., margarine, shortening, cooking spray and all hydrogenated or partially hydrogenated oils).

2. Eat animal fats in moderation (i.e., eggs, steak, yogurt, etc.). Use common sense. Too much meat or animal protein can contribute to high cholesterol and other diseases. On the other hand, completely avoiding these things may only aggravate you and cause emotional stress, which is likely a bigger factor in heart disease than animal fats.

3. Start taking essential fatty acid supplements such as cod liver oil and omega-3, -6 and -9 supplements. Consult with a healthcare practitioner before taking dietary supplements and about the possibility of reducing your cholesterol medication.

4. Eat vegetables in all their varieties and in the seasons they ripen. Include plenty of whole-grain foods in your diet, and don't be fooled by packaged, processed products that tout heart health.

Recommended supplements:

Lipid Systemic Enzyme
PhytoNutrient
KardiGen™*

*From a company in Singapore (see www.kardigen.com).

Cold, Fevers, Flu

Conventional wisdom suggests that there is no cure for the common cold. This is true, as colds are caused by a depressed immune system succumbing to a virus of the immune system, but there are proper ways to treat cold symptoms. Unfortunately, most cold suppressants just mask the symptoms and never address the cause.

A common saying in the herbal industry is, "Feed a cold and starve a fever." Simply put, nourish those with a cold and give only liquids to those with a fever. Allow fevers to run their course. A fever is the body's defense mechanism against a viral or bacterial infection. Intervene with medication when a fever is high or has persisted for several hours. When you feel tired, get some rest. If you feel congested, let the body drain. Don't suppress symptoms with medications unless the symptoms become intolerable or life threatening.

One of the worst mistakes most people make while treating a fever is providing nourishment to the body. The quickest way to get over a fever is to fast. Drink plenty of water and juice but don't waste your energy on digestion; let your body use that energy for building the immune system to fight the virus. Once the fever has passed, eat easily digested foods like soups or fresh fruit.

The following natural antibiotic has been effective for a cold or fever. I have used this infusion for strep throat, fevers or colds.

Use four cups of apple juice instead of water for taste, and make an infusion of the following:

     2 crushed garlic bulbs

     1 oz. chopped lemongrass

     2 teaspoons oregano oil (herbal oil)

     2 tablespoons raw honey

Simmer (do not boil) the apple juice, garlic and lemongrass

for 20 minutes. Then add the oregano oil and raw honey. Stir to melt the honey and then pour one cup through a strainer to drink. Put the strained garlic and lemongrass back into the remaining three cups of apple juice. Every three hours, reheat the remaining liquid and drink one cup. This will give you 12 hours of natural antibiotics. Usually the cold will be gone by the next day. If not, repeat this process.

If your cold includes a sore throat, you can omit the oregano oil and instead add one teaspoon of cayenne pepper to the mixture. My grandmother called this "firewater," and it was constantly brewed in my childhood home with seven children. I use it today for my kids, and my neighbors have begun to knock on my door at all hours of the night asking me to brew it for them as well.

Colic

In adults, biliary colic is caused by a blockage in the gallbladder, bile duct or cystic duct. It is commonly caused by gallstones getting stuck in the cystic or bile duct resulting in severe pain in the upper abdomen.

Make an infusion of the following:

1 oz. peppermint leaves	1 slice of lemon
1 tablespoon raw honey	1 pint of water or juice

Sip as needed while infusion is warm. Reheat if it cools.

Because it contains honey, do not give this infusion to infants or children under the age of one. Honey can harbor dormant bacteria that cause botulism and the digestive tracts of children are not sufficiently developed to destroy the bacteria.

Many infants experience a form of colic, which is diagnosed when a healthy baby frequently cries without any discernible reason.

Rooibos tea is a good way to relieve colic in infants. Make the tea and let it cool until lukewarm. Put the tea into the baby's bottle and allow the baby to drink as much as desired. Another good remedy is a warm bath.

Colon Care (irritable bowel syndrome, diverticulitis, colitis and other colon problems)

Dry and grind into powder the following herbs:

> 200 grams fenugreek seeds
> 100 grams comfrey leaves and root
> 200 grams acacia gum
> 300 grams psyllium seed husks
> 300 grams goldenseal root
> 100 grams myrrh gum

Mix well and encapsulate into 1,000 mg (size 00) capsules. Take four of these capsules every day for four weeks. A bloated feeling is natural for about 10 days. Continue if problem persists. Eat lots of fiber and drink slippery elm tea to allow for healing after this therapy.

Note: Due to its pyrrolizidine alkaloid content, people with liver problems should avoid taking comfrey internally. People with high blood pressure or liver disease should avoid goldenseal.

Recommended supplements:

Total Body Detox
Total Systemic Enzyme

Constipation

Make a decoction of the following:

> 1 oz. cascara sagrada bark
> 1/2 oz. raspberry leaves
> 1/2 oz. flaxseeds
> 1/2 oz. rhubarb stalk (rhubarb leaves are toxic)

Bring one quart of water to a boil and add the herbs. Turn down the heat and let it simmer for 30 minutes. Strain the liquid and drink one cup every hour until relieved.

Another way to get a quick bowel movement is to add 1/2 cup of sea salt to one pint of warm water. Drink it all. This will cause a gallbladder bile flush, and within one hour you will need to visit the restroom.

You can prevent constipation by drinking plenty of pure water and eating a diet high in whole grains and vegetables. If you suffer from chronic constipation, I advise you to visit a colon hydrotherapist and make changes in your diet.

Recommended supplements:

Total Systemic Enzyme
Total Body Detox

Coughs

A decoction of the following makes a great natural cough syrup remedy:

> 1/2 oz. horehound root
> 1/2 oz. elecampane root
> 1/2 oz. comfrey root
> 1/2 oz. wild cherry bark

Boil combination in two quarts of water until there is only one quart left. Strain the herbs out and add six to eight ounces of honey. Take a tablespoon of this every half an hour as needed.

Note: Due to its pyrrolizidine alkaloid content, people with liver problems should avoid taking comfrey internally.

While trying to get rid of a cough or a sore throat, do not consume any dairy products. Also try a deep breathing exercise of sucking in air for seven seconds, holding in for seven seconds, and letting out for seven seconds. Try this for five minutes in the morning and five minutes before bedtime.

Diabetes (Type 1)

Type 1 diabetes is a blood sugar disorder that occurs when the body does not produce sufficient insulin to properly process the carbohydrates and sugar an individual consumes. At this present time and with present knowledge, type 1 diabetes is incurable. (When I say "incurable," I mean with present scientific knowledge. I truly believe that the body knows how to cure all things, and that with proper nutrients, rest and faith, all things are possible. There has been much headway in stem cell research. This research shows a lot of promise for people with type 1 diabetes.)

However, life expectancy and quality of life can be greatly improved by using alternative treatments. The following actions are recommended to ensure quality of life for people with type 1 diabetes.

1. Brush skin daily. Buy a dry skin brush at a health food store and brush the skin before showering each day. Brush in a circular motion starting at the tips of the extremities and always working your way toward the heart. This allows for

increased circulation to the extremities, ensuring proper nerve function.

2. Take oligomeric proanthocyanidin (OPC) antioxidants daily. OPC antioxidants—found in grapeseed extract, maritime pine bark, bilberry and other sources—are particularly powerful antioxidants that may provide support for stabilizing blood sugar levels. Red blood cells, veins, arteries and capillary cells need to stay soft and pliable in order to function properly. Free radicals can cause these cells to become hard and brittle. OPCs and other antioxidants may help keep cells soft and pliable by limiting free radical damage. By reducing free radical damage and potentially softening cells, OPC antioxidants may provide support for glaucoma and macular degeneration for people with type 1 diabetes.

3. Drink one cup of dandelion root tea or cedar berry tea every day. These herbs support proper kidney function and can extend the life of the kidneys.

4. Drink huckleberry leaf tea three times a week. This tea feeds the pancreas and improves digestion.

5. Take digestive enzymes with each meal. Predigesting sugars before they enter the bloodstream helps the body process those sugars more efficiently. People who do this are sometimes able to cut back on their intake of insulin, thus preserving the liver and kidneys.

Recommended supplements:

PhytoNutrient
All Omega Fat Complex
Total Systemic Enzyme

Diabetes (Type 2)

Not only is type 2 diabetes treatable, but in many cases its effects can be reversed. It takes discipline and education to accomplish this. Correcting bad eating habits is the first step to reversing the problem.

Two problems are associated with type 2 diabetes. The first problem is insulin resistance, in which insulin receptors in the cells become unresponsive to insulin. The second problem is improper insulin-sugar balance, which occurs when one eats so much sugar (carbohydrates) that the body cannot produce enough insulin to process the excess.

1. Stop eating processed carbohydrates, such as white flour, sugar, candy, potato chips and soft drinks.

2. Follow a diet high in raw plant proteins. Many physicians believe that an increase of protein content will eventually lead to kidney stones, rheumatoid arthritis and gout. They are right, if the protein comes from meat. However, if one's protein comes from raw, predominantly plant sources, this will not happen. Uricase is an enzyme found in raw protein sources that breaks down urates (a byproduct of protein digestion), allowing the body to eliminate monosodium urate and preventing many problems associated with high-protein diets.

3. Eat lots of green fibrous vegetables like asparagus, celery and broccoli. Though these are carbohydrates, they will not cause your blood sugar to spike.

4. Take systemic enzyme supplements.

5. Sprout seeds and eats lots of them.

6. Avoid dairy foods.

People with type 2 diabetes can also benefit from the advice given to people with type 1 diabetes on pages 95–96. Doing these things may help your blood sugar come down, saving a lot of future problems.

Recommended supplements:

PhytoNutrient
All Omega Fat Complex
Total Systemic Enzyme

Diarrhea and Dysentery

Oatmeal is a natural treatment for diarrhea. Eat one cup of cooked oatmeal once every two hours until the condition has improved. Slippery elm bark tea can also help, but it takes several hours for it to work.

Don't forget to drink plenty of pure, filtered water (not juice) during and after this condition. Diarrhea is a symptom of the body trying to get rid of something. Let this happen, but don't let yourself become dehydrated.

Gout

Internal

In two quarts of water or apple juice, make a decoction of:

2 oz. chaparral leaf	1/2 oz. burdock root
1 oz. yucca root	1/2 oz. black cohosh root
1/2 oz. dandelion roots	1/2 oz. ginger root
1/2 oz. prickly ash bark	

Drink six ounces of this decoction three times a day for about two weeks. It will lower uric acid levels in the blood and begin to reduce the amount of inflammation. (Uric acid is produced as the body breaks down meats and high fat dairy products like ice cream. In excess, it can accumulate in the joints, causing pain and inflammation.) This decoction also nourishes the thymus, which balances white blood cell production. In an attack of gout, the body overproduces white blood cells.

Note: Due to potential for liver damage, the FDA cautions against the internal use of chaparral.

Topically (for pain)
Make a liniment of:

> 1 pint rubbing alcohol
> 1/2 oz. oil of eucalyptus (herbal oil)
> 1/2 oz. oil of wintergreen (herbal oil)

Recommended eating:

Avoid any foods that will raise uric acid levels in the blood. These include meat and dairy products, carbonated drinks, alcohol and coffee. Help your body lower acid levels by drinking lots of filtered water, eating lots of leafy vegetables (at least five servings a day) and consider fasting for 12 hours at least once a week.

Hay Fever (or allergies with similar symptoms)

Make an infusion of the following:

> 1 oz. Brigham tea (see page 77)
> 1/2 oz. sage leaves (fresh)
> 1/2 oz. ginger root (chopped)
> 1 quart water

Beginning a few weeks before allergy season, drink one cup once a day, then drink several times daily as needed for symptoms. It won't be long before symptoms disappear completely.

Recommended supplements:

Immune Modulating Complex

Headache

Make an infusion of the following:

> 1 oz. skullcap leaves
> 1 oz. rosemary leaves
> 1 oz. peppermint leaves or flowers
> 1 oz. chamomile flowers
> 1 tablespoon raw honey for flavor
> 1 quart water or apple juice

Drink one cup as needed.

If the headache is a tension headache, you may get relief by pressing hard with your thumb or middle finger into the lower neck or upper shoulder area for 10 minutes, or have someone do it for you. You can determine whether a headache is a tension headache by pressing hard with your finger into the upper shoulder. If there is pain, then most likely it is a tension headache.

Recommended supplements:

Herbal Calming Blend

Infections

Most infections can be treated with natural antibiotics such as the following:

> garlic, lemongrass, juniper berries, dandelion roots, oregano oil, thyme, sage leaves, cloves, ginger, horseradish and coneflower root (*Echinacea*)

These natural antibiotics can be eaten during an illness or infection or applied topically to skin infections. They may also be used in a decoction or infusion in any quantity. *Remember that with all antibiotic herbs you should not use the same ones over and over.* Eventually, bacteria will adapt and overcome. Switch the type of herb or food you are using with each infection to avoid creating a resistance to a particular antibiotic herb. If your infection worsens or does not improve, see a healthcare practitioner.

Recommended supplements:

ViraGuard

Insomnia

Before treating insomnia with herbs, be sure you are not just worried or stressed about work, kids, finances, etc. If your mind is not at peace, you will not be able to sleep well. This can lead to premature aging, inability to heal wounds or organs properly and emotional mood swings. Meditate or pray to clear your mind. Breathe deeply and listen only to your breathing for a few minutes. If you still cannot sleep after trying those things, try supporting insomnia with herbs.

Make an infusion of the following:

> 1 oz. catnip leaves
>
> 1 oz. chamomile leaves
>
> 1 oz. valerian root
>
> 1 oz. peppermint leaves

Steep for 10 minutes in one quart of hot water, strain and sweeten with honey to taste. Drink one or two cups and the sheep will appear out of nowhere in 15–20 minutes.

Recommended supplements:

Herbal Calming Blend

Menopause

Make an infusion or decoction of the following:

> 2 oz. black cohosh root
>
> 1 oz. red raspberry leaves
>
> 1 oz. false unicorn root
>
> 1 oz. licorice root
>
> 1 oz. ginger

Steep for 10 minutes in one quart of hot water, strain and sweeten with raw honey to taste. Drink one cup in the morning and two cups in the evening.

Recommended eating:

Supplement your diet with highly nutrient-dense foods such as kelp, dulse, other sea greens and broccoli for calcium. Also include foods that contain plant-based estrogen such as soy products (soy milk, edamame, tofu, etc.), strawberries, sweet potatoes, raspberries and cucumbers. These will all assist in making menopausal years easier to deal with emotionally and help prevent estrogen-related degenerative diseases such as osteoporosis and breast, uterine, ovarian and cervical cancers.

Recommended supplements:

Complete Phytoestrogens
All Omega Fat Complex

Menstruation (pain/cramping or heavy bleeding)

Make a decoction of the following:

> 1 oz. cramp bark
> 1 oz. skullcap leaves
> 1 oz. false unicorn root
> a pinch of cayenne powder

Steep for 10 minutes in one quart of hot water, strain and sweeten with raw honey to taste. Drink one pint a day during the week prior to your period. This decoction should help alleviate cramping or heavy bleeding.

Recommended supplements:

Complete Phytoestrogens

Morning Sickness

Make an infusion of the following:

> 2 oz. red raspberry leaves
> 1 oz. lemon peels (pesticide free)
> 1 oz. ginger root

Steep for 10 minutes in one quart of hot water and strain. Sweeten with one tablespoon raw honey. Drink as needed.

Recommended supplements:

The Works™
Total Systemic Enzyme

Obesity

Finally recognized as a major problem in the United States, obesity affects nearly every household and costs taxpayers hundreds of thousands of dollars every year in subsidized insurance premiums and healthcare costs.

The major cause of this problem is not glandular (i.e., thyroid problems, hormonal changes, etc.). It is the portion size, frequency and types of food we eat. I once watched a woman consume three slices of cheesecake in the time it took me to eat half of one. What a sugar rush! Imagine 140 grams of carbohydrates—more than half the amount recommended for an entire day—flooding the body within 10 minutes! It's no wonder that obesity is such a pervasive problem in the U.S.

Recommended lifestyle changes

It may take months to achieve your goal, but the weight will come off if you follow these steps.

1. Eat a variety of foods in small portions. My typical breakfast includes a boiled egg, a small bowl of oatmeal, a carrot slice, a cucumber slice and a quarter of an apple. As you increase the variety of foods in your meals, you will feel more satisfied—and you may save some money on grocery bills!

2. Shop on the edges of the grocery store, not the aisles.

The edges include the dairy section, the produce section, the meat section, the bakery and the deli. These sections contain the fresh and real food (enzyme-rich cheeses, fresh meat, fresh fruits and vegetables). The aisles contain packaged, preservative-rich, low-nutrient foods that we can do without.

3. At each meal, fill half your plate with vegetables of any kind in a variety of colors, and a quarter of your plate with meat or complex carbohydrates like beans or brown rice. If you are not satisfied after eating, fill the remaining quarter of your plate with another helping of vegetables.

4. Eat only until you are satisfied, not until you are full.

5. Avoid fad diets or any diet that tells you to limit your food variety (i.e., juice diet, grapefruit diet, banana diet, etc.).

6. *Do not use herbal stimulants* unless you have been diagnosed with hypothyroidism, in which case use them only in the morning. Otherwise they can become addictive, which can further harm your glandular system.

7. Eat lots of sea greens or take kelp capsules.

8. Drink plenty of pure, filtered water (try to drink half your body weight in ounces daily—75 oz. for a 150 lb. person).

9. Take digestive enzymes with each meal.

Parasites

The immune system protects us from most of the harmful parasites in the broader meaning of the word. We all have parasites, but most are not harmful. If you are diagnosed with a harmful parasite, the following herbs may be helpful.

Make a decoction of:

> 2 oz. wormwood bark
>
> 2 oz. crushed garlic bulbs
>
> 2 oz. black walnut hulls
>
> 1 oz. oregano leaves

Bring one quart of water to a boil and add the herbs. Turn down the heat and let it simmer for 30 minutes. Strain the liquid and flavor with lemon juice. Drink one cup three times a day.

Avoid any excessively sweet foods during this treatment. (See also Cold, Fevers, Flu on page 90 and Infections on page 101, as the treatments recommended in these sections also contain many antifungal and antiparasitic agents.)

Recommended supplements:

ViraGuard

Immune Modulating Complex

Skin Conditions (eczema, psoriasis, dryness and itchiness)

Make an herbal oil containing the following:

> 2 oz. calendula blossoms   1 oz. St. John's wort
>
> 2 oz. plantain leaves   1 oz. chamomile leaves
>
> 2 oz. chickweed

Apply or massage the oil onto dry areas three times daily. It may also be helpful to purchase a real plant fiber exfoliation brush or a real sponge and dry brush and exfoliate up to three times a day.

Eat foods that are high in sodium, sulfur and magnesium such as peaches, almonds, kelp, garlic, grapes, celery, spinach, goat's milk, apricots, papaya and melons.

For itchy skin and rashes due to eczema, psoriasis or allergies, the following can help greatly. Combine the following ingredients into a bowl:

> 3/4 cup aloe vera gel
> 2 tablespoons blended oats or oat flour
> 15 drops tea tree oil
> 1/2 tablespoon calendula leaves

Mix together well and place in a jar after adding some vitamin E or lemon juice as a preservative. This really soothes itchiness. Other herbs like lavender flowers, chamomile leaves or rose hip seed powder can be added as preservative and fragrance enhancers as well.

For skin that's dry simply due to dryness of the air, frequent changes in climate or after swimming or bathing, this simple formula for a common lotion may be used to moisturize your skin completely:

> 1/3 cup coconut oil
> 2 tablespoons olive oil
> 1 tablespoon emulsifying
>   wax or beeswax
> 1/8 teaspoon lecithin
> 1/2 cup water

> 1/2 cup aloe vera gel
> a few drops of an
>   essential oil or other
>   herbs as desired (I have
>   found that lavender
>   oil works best)

Blend the coconut oil, olive oil, wax and lecithin in a double boiler, heating just enough to melt and mix the ingredients. Add 1/2 cup boiling water and stir thoroughly. When the mixture cools to room temperature, add 1/2 cup aloe vera gel. Mix well by hand or with a hand blender, then add the essential oils/herbs.

Try various essential oils to give the lotion the fragrance you desire. An essential oil with high antioxidant activity can also act as a preservative.

Stomach Ache (nausea, cramping, indigestion)

Make an infusion of the following:

>   2 oz. ginger root (chopped)
>   2 oz. peppermint leaves

Steep for 10 minutes in one quart of hot water, strain and sweeten with raw honey to taste. Drink one cup every 30 minutes. Sometimes eating half a cup of yogurt with enzyme cultures helps as well.

Ulcers

Make a decoction of the following:

>   1 oz. slippery elm bark
>   1 oz. marshmallow root
>   1 oz. goldenseal root
>   1 oz. licorice root

Bring one quart of water to a boil and add the herbs. Turn down the heat and let simmer for 30 minutes. Strain the liquid. Drink one cup in the evening and one in the morning for one week.

Note: People with high blood pressure or liver disease should avoid goldenseal.

During this time, try to find a good source of a liquid trace mineral drink and take one ounce once a day. Certain trace minerals may help kill the bacteria that cause ulcers. In a study published in 2006 in the *Trakia Journal of Sciences*, researchers found that copper and selenium reduced ulcers in pig tissue, which is similar to human tissue.

We should all be getting a variety of trace minerals from vegetables. However, some vegetables can become depleted of minerals and fail to provide sufficient amounts. I use the trace minerals from Organa Mineral Products, Inc. I have personally tested them for heavy metal content as well as amino acids (which should be found in any organic trace mineral complex).

Virus-Related Fevers (measles, chicken pox, smallpox, etc.)

For topical treatment of the sores, itchiness or rashes, make a strong decoction of thyme and cloves. Soak a towel in the decoction and apply to the skin several times daily.

For internal treatment, make an infusion of the following:

> 1 oz. calendula blossoms
> 1 oz. yarrow root (diced)
> 1 oz. red onion (diced)
> raw honey or xylitol to flavor

Steep herbs in one quart of hot water for 10 minutes and strain. Drink one cup every three hours. In addition, drink diluted juices such as lemon, lime, grapefruit and carrot juices throughout the day.

Ingredients in Recommended Supplements

Ingredients in the recommended NutraNomics® formulas are listed as follows. I formulated these products and believe in their effectiveness; however, if you find products that you prefer that contain similar ingredients, feel free to substitute.

All Omega Fat Complex: An essential fatty acid supplement that contains vitamin E, flax oil, borage oil and fish oil (providing omega-3, -6, and -9).

Complete Phytoestrogens: A phytoestrogen supplement that contains saw palmetto, *Angelica sinensis*, damiana leaf powder, blessed thistle, licorice root, wild yam, motherwort, black cohosh root, red raspberry leaf, false unicorn powder, passion flower, cramp bark and dong quai root.

Herbal Calming Blend: A calming supplement that contains valerian root, chamomile flower, lavender flower, passion flower, peppermint leaves powder, hops flower extract, catnip, skullcap powder, bacopa (*Bacopa monnieri*), myrrh gum and feverfew leaves.

Immune Modulating Complex: An immune supporting supplement that contains cat's claw (*Uncaria tomentosa*), Oregon grape (*Mahonia aquifolium*), astragalus, cranberry powder, reishi mushroom, aloe vera, maitake mushroom and royal jelly.

Lipid Systemic Enzyme: A fat digestion supplement that contains protease, amylase, lipase, cellulase, kelp, coral calcium, magnesium citrate, zinc gluconate, manganese gluconate, pectin and HCl.

PhytoNutrient: An antioxidant supplement that contains red grape extract, pomegranate extract, mangosteen powder, broccoli powder, cocoa powder, bilberry extract, grapefruit extract, tomato powder, carrot powder concentrate and raspberry leaf.

Total Systemic Enzyme: A digestive enzyme complex that contains protease, amylase, cellulase, sucrase, maltase, lactase, coral calcium and kelp.

ViraGuard: An infection-fighting supplement that contains pau d'arco, garlic powder, olive leaf extract, black walnut hulls, sarsaparilla root powder, cloves powder and *Artemisia annua* (wormwood) leaves.

The Works™: A multivitamin complex that contains vitamin A, B-complex, C, D₃, E, coral calcium, magnesium, iron, zinc, manganese, selenium, chromium, barley grass, alfalfa leaf, chlorella, sunflower seed, catnip, acerola cherry and 72 trace minerals.

Herb-Drug
Contraindications

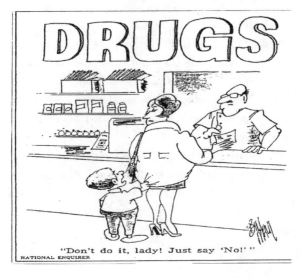

"Don't do it, lady! Just say 'No!'"

NATIONAL ENQUIRER

For this chapter, I have compiled an alphabetical list of the most commonly prescribed drugs and added to it my thoughts on herbs that should not be used if you have chosen to take those particular medications. Taking prescription drugs is *your choice*. Find a doctor who is open-minded and willing to work with you in finding the best treatments for your specific ailments.

My purpose in creating this list is to assist you and your doctor in watching for possible contraindications in case you are taking a prescription or OTC drug. These potential contraindications are not necessarily deadly. Remember that all of these drugs remain in the bloodstream for different amounts of time, and the contraindications I list below only apply to the use of the herb while the drug is actively in the bloodstream. In other words, if you took a Tylenol for a headache, it would be best to not take feverfew for the next six to eight hours. However, after the drug has left the bloodstream, it would be fine to take feverfew. *It is quite possible that the use of these herbs while taking the drug would cause no reaction, but based on my experience and knowledge of the active phytochemicals that may or may not be found in an herb, depending on how it was harvested and processed, it is safer not to use it.*

In the following chart, the pharmaceutical drugs are listed in bold, followed by herbal contraindications. I have created this list for safety reasons. Always consult with a healthcare practitioner before mixing prescriptions medications and herbal remedies.

Abciximab (Reopro®) Avoid supplements containing feverfew (*Tanacetum parthenium*), garlic (*Allium sativum*), *Ginkgo biloba* or ginger (*Zingiber officinale*).

ACE inhibitors (Captopril®, Enalapril®) Avoid supplements containing 2,000 mg or more of potassium or yohimbe (*Pausinystalia yohimbe*).

Acetaminophen (Tylenol®) Avoid supplements containing more than one gram of evening primrose oil (*Oenothera biennis*) or any amount of feverfew (*Tanacetum parthenium*).

Acetylsalicylic acid (Ecotrin®) Avoid supplements containing feverfew (*Tanacetum parthenium*).

Acular® (ketorolac) Avoid supplements containing gossypol (*Gossypium hirsutum*), one gram or more of white willow (*Salix* species) or feverfew (*Tanacetum parthenium*).

Adriamycin® (doxorubicin) Avoid supplements containing more than 250 mg of St. John's wort (*Hypericum perforatum*).

Agrylin® (Anagrelide HCl) Avoid supplements containing any feverfew (*Tanacetum parthenium*), large amounts of garlic (*Allium sativum*), ginger (*Zingiber officinale*) or one gram or more of *Ginkgo biloba*.

Akineton® (Biperiden) Avoid supplements containing betel nut (*Piper betle*), mandrake (*Mandragora officinarum*) or jimson weed (*Datura stramonium*) a.k.a. thornapple.

Aldactone® (spironolactone) Avoid supplements containing licorice (*Glycyrrhiza glabra*) or large amounts of potassium (2,000 mg or more).

Aldomet® (methyldopa) Avoid supplements containing 10 mg or more of iron.

Alora® (estradiol) Avoid supplements containing 500 mg or more of ginseng (*Panax ginseng*), *Hoodia* or any human growth hormones.

Alprazolam (Xanax®) Avoid supplements containing any kava kava (*Piper methysticum*), false unicorn (*Chamaelirium luteum*) or chamomile.

Alteplase (Activase®) Avoid supplements containing any feverfew (*Tanacetum parthenium*) one gram or more of garlic (*Allium sativum*), *Ginkgo biloba* or ginger (*Zingiber officinale*).

Amantadine HCl (Symmetrel®)   Avoid supplements containing 250 mg or more of chasteberry (*Vitex agnus-castus*) or Oregon grape (*Mahonia aquifolium*).

Amiloride HCI (Midamor®, Moduretic®)   Avoid supplements containing 500 mg or more of licorice root (*Glycyrrhiza glabra*) or potassium.

Aminophylline® (theophylline)   Salicylates interfere with absorption of Aminophylline® when taken simultaneously. Thus, avoid meadowsweet herb (*Filipendula ulmaria*), poplar herb (*Populus* species), 500 mg or more of white willow bark (*Salix* species), or wintergreen (*Gaultheria procumbens, Pyrola rotundifolia*). Herbs high in tannins also impair absorption if taken simultaneously, so avoid green or black tea (*Camellia sinensis*), uva ursi (*Arctostaphylos uva-ursi*), black walnut (*Juglans nigra*), red raspberry (*Rubus idaeus*), oak (*Quercus robur*) or witch hazel (*Hamamelis virginiana*).

Amiodarone (Cordarone®, Pacerone®)   Avoid supplements containing *Echinacea* species, licorice (*Glycyrrhiza glabra*) or cascara sagrada (*Rhamnus purshianus*).

Amnesteem®, formerly known as Accutane® (isotretinoin)   Avoid supplements containing high amounts (25,000 IU or higher) of vitamin A.

Anafranil® (clomipramine HCl)   Avoid supplements containing St. John's wort (*Hypericum perforatum*).

Anagrelide HCl (Agrylin®)   Avoid supplements containing any feverfew (*Tanacetum parthenium*), large amounts of garlic (*Allium sativum*), ginger (*Zingiber officinale*) or one gram or more of *Ginkgo biloba*.

Anaprox® (naproxen)   Avoid supplements containing feverfew (*Tanacetum parthenium*).

Ardeparin sodium (Normiflo®)   Avoid supplements containing feverfew (*Tanacetum parthenium*), garlic (*Allium sativum*), *Ginkgo biloba* or ginger (*Zingiber officinale*).

Aricept® (donepezil)   Avoid supplements containing betel nut (*Piper betle*), mandrake (*Mandragora officinarum*) or jimson weed (*Datura stramonium*) a.k.a. thornapple.

Arthrotec® (diclofenac, misoprostol)   Avoid supplements containing feverfew (*Tanacetum parthenium*), gossypol (*Gossypium hirsutum*) and white willow (*Salix* species).

Atamet® (carbidopa)   Avoid supplements containing iron or kava kava (*Piper methysticum*).

Ativan® (benzodiazepene)   Avoid supplements containing kava kava (*Piper methysticum*).

Atropine sulfate   Avoid supplements containing 500 mg or more of white willow bark (*Salix* species) or wintergreen (*Gaultheria procumbens; Pyrola rotundifolia*). Also avoid tannins, such as green or black tea (*Camellia sinensis*), uva ursi (*Arctostaphylos uva-ursi*), black walnut (*Juglans nigra*), red raspberry (*Rubus idaeus*), oak (*Quercus robur*) and witch hazel (*Hamamelis virginiana*).

Atrovent® (ipratropium)   Avoid supplements containing betel nut (*Piper betle*), mandrake (*Mandragora officinarum*) or jimson weed (*Datura stramonium*) a.k.a. thornapple.

Azathioprine (Imuran®)   Avoid supplements containing andrographis (*Andrographis paniculata*), ashwagandha (*Withania somnifera*), *Astragalus* species, *Echinacea* species, garlic (*Allium sativum*), ginseng (*Panax ginseng*), maitake (*Grifola frondosa*), reishi (*Ganoderma lucidum*), magnolia vine (*Schisandra chinensis*) or suma (*Pfaffia paniculata*).

Bactrim® (trimethoprim, sulfamethoxazole)   Avoid supplements containing potassium.

Basiliximab (Simulect®)   Avoid supplements containing andrographis (*Andrographis paniculata*), ashwagandha (*Withania somnifera*), *Astragalus* species, *Echinacea* species, garlic (*Allium sativum*), ginseng (*Panax ginseng*), maitake (*Grifola frondosa*), reishi (*Ganoderma lucidum*), magnolia vine (*Schisandra chinensis*) or suma (*Pfaffia paniculata*).

Benzodiazepene (Ativan®)   Avoid supplements containing kava kava (*Piper methysticum*).

Benztropine (Cogentin®)   Avoid supplements containing betel nut (*Piper betle*), mandrake (*Mandragora officinarum*) or jimson weed (*Datura stramonium*) a.k.a. thornapple.

Betamethasone (Celestone®, Diprolene®, Lotrisone®) Avoid supplements containing licorice (*Glycyrrhiza glabra*), magnolia bark (*Magnolia officinalis*), perilla (*Perilla frutescens*), Saiboku-to (a Japanese 5-herb bupleurum decoction), Baikal skullcap (*Scutellaria baicalensis*) or jujube (*Ziziphus vulgaris*).

Betapace® (sotalol) Avoid supplements containing licorice (*Glycyrrhiza glabra*) or cascara sagrada (*Rhamnus purshianus*).

Bethanechol (Urecholine®) Avoid supplements containing betel nut (*Piper betle*), mandrake (*Mandragora officinarum*) or jimson weed (*Datura stramonium*) a.k.a. thornapple.

Biperiden (Akineton®) Avoid supplements containing 500 mg or more of betel nut (*Piper betle*), mandrake (*Mandragora officinarum*) or jimson weed (*Datura stramonium*) a.k.a. thornapple.

Bromocriptine (Parlodel®) Avoid supplements containing chasteberry (*Vitex agnus-castus*).

Bumetanide (Bumex®) Avoid supplements containing licorice (*Glycyrrhiza glabra*), ginseng (*Panax ginseng*), germanium (Ge-Oxy 132) or gossypol (*Gossypium hirsutum*).

Bumex® (bumetanide) Avoid supplements containing licorice (*Glycyrrhiza glabra*), ginseng (*Panax ginseng*), germanium (Ge-Oxy 132) or gossypol (*Gossypium hirsutum*).

Calan® (verapamil) Avoid supplements containing calcium, licorice (*Glycyrrhiza glabra*) or cascara sagrada (*Rhamnus purshianus*).

Captopril® (ACE inhibitor) Avoid supplements containing 2,000 mg or more of potassium or yohimbe (*Pausinystalia yohimbe*).

Carafate® (sucralfate) May bind to herbal supplements, thereby preventing absorption.

Carbamazepine (Carbatrol®, Tegretol®) Avoid supplements containing *Ginkgo biloba*.

Carbidopa (Atamet®, Sinemet®) Avoid supplements containing iron or kava kava (*Piper methysticum*).

Cataflam® (diclofenac, misoprostol) Avoid supplements containing fever-few (*Tanacetum parthenium*).

Catapres® (clonidine HCl) Avoid supplements containing yohimbe (*Pausinystalia yohimbe*).

Celestone® (betamethasone) Avoid supplements containing licorice (*Glycyrrhiza glabra*), magnolia bark (*Magnolia officinalis*), perilla (*Perilla frutescens*), Saiboku-to, Baikal skullcap (*Scutellaria baicalensis*) or jujube (*Ziziphus vulgaris*).

Chlorodiazepoxide (Librium®) Avoid supplements containing kava kava (*Piper methysticum*).

Chlorpromazine (Thorazine®) Avoid supplements containing chasteberry (*Vitex agnus-castus*) or kava kava (*Piper methysticum*).

Chlorpropamide (Diabinese®) Avoid supplements containing bilberry (*Vaccinium myrtillus*), bitter melon (*Momordica charantia*), ivy gourd (*Coccinia indica*), garlic (*Allium sativum*), ginseng (*Panax ginseng*), gurmar (*Gymnema sylvestre*), onion (*Allium cepa*), Indian kino (*Pterocarpus marsupium*), jambul (*Syzygium cumini*), fenugreek (*Trigonella foenum-graecum*) or salt bush (*Atriplex halimus*).

Chlorthiazide (Diuril®) Avoid supplements containing licorice (*Glycyrrhiza glabra*).

Cholestyramine (Questran®) May bind to herbal supplements, thereby preventing absorption.

Cipro® (ciproflaxacin) Avoid supplements containing iron, calcium or zinc.

Clinoril® (sulindac) Avoid supplements containing feverfew (*Tanacetum parthenium*).

Clomipramine HCl (Anafranil®) Avoid supplements containing St. John's wort (*Hypericum perforatum*).

Clonidine HCl (Catapres®, Clorpres®, Combipres®, Duraclon®) Avoid supplements containing yohimbe (*Pausinystalia yohimbe*).

Clopidogrel (Plavix®) Avoid supplements containing feverfew (*Tanacetum parthenium*), garlic (*Allium sativum*), *Ginkgo biloba* or ginger (*Zingiber officinale*).

Clorazepate (Tranxene®, Gen-XENE®) Avoid supplements containing kava kava (*Piper methysticum*).

Clozapine (Clozaril®) Avoid supplements containing St. John's wort (*Hypericum perforatum*).

Codeine Avoid herbs containing salicylates. Avoid herbs high in tannins. (*See listing for aminophylline on page 116 for more details.*)

Cogentin® (benztropine) Avoid supplements containing betel nut (*Piper betle*), mandrake (*Mandragora officinarum*) or jimson weed (*Datura stramonium*) a.k.a. thornapple.

Colestid® (colestipol) May bind to herbal supplements, thereby preventing absorption.

Combipres® (clonidine HCl) Avoid supplements containing yohimbe (*Pausinystalia yohimbe*).

Combivent® (Ipratropium) Avoid supplements containing betel nut (*Piper betle*), mandrake (*Mandragora officinarum*) or jimson weed (*Datura stramonium*) a.k.a. thornapple.

Compazine® (prochlorperazine) Avoid supplements containing evening primrose oil (*Oenothera biennis*).

Cordarone® (amiodarone) Avoid supplements containing *Echinacea* species, licorice (*Glycyrrhiza glabra*) or cascara sagrada (*Rhamnus purshianus*).

Coumadin (Warfarin®) Avoid supplements containing vitamin K, coenzyme Q10, vitamin D, vitamin E, vitamin C, bromelain, danshen (*Salvia miltiorrhiza*), garlic (*Allium sativum*), feverfew (*Tanacetum parthenium*), ginseng (*Panax ginseng*), ginger (*Zingiber officinale*), dong quai root (*Angelica sinensis*), *Ginkgo biloba* or vinpocetine.

Crixivan® (Indinavir) Avoid supplements containing St. John's wort (*Hypericum perforatum*).

Cuprimine® (penicillamine) Avoid supplements containing copper or iron.

Cyclosporine (Neoral®, Sandimmune®)   Avoid supplements containing *Echinacea* species and St. John's wort (*Hypericum perforatum*).

Daclizumab (Zenapax®)   Avoid supplements containing andrographis (*Andrographis paniculata*), ashwagandha *(Withania somnifera)*, *Astragalus* species, *Echinacea* species, garlic (*Allium sativum*), ginseng (*Panax ginseng*), maitake (*Grifola frondosa*), reishi (*Ganoderma lucidum*), magnolia vine (*Schisandra chinensis*) or suma (*Pfaffia paniculata*).

Dalteparin (Fragmin®)   Avoid supplements containing feverfew (*Tanacetum parthenium*), garlic (*Allium sativum*), *Ginkgo biloba* or ginger (*Zingiber officinale*).

Danaparoid (Orgaran®)   Avoid supplements containing feverfew (*Tanacetum parthenium*), garlic (*Allium sativum*), *Ginkgo biloba* or ginger (*Zingiber officinale*).

Daypro® (oxaprozin)   Avoid supplements containing feverfew (*Tanacetum parthenium*).

Depen® (penicillamine)   Avoid supplements containing copper or iron.

Desferal® (deferoxamine)   Avoid supplements containing iron.

Dexamethasone (Decadron®, Decaspray®, TobraDex®, Dalalone D.P.®, Dexacort®, NeoDecadron®)   Avoid supplements containing licorice (*Glycyrrhiza glabra*), magnolia bark (*Magnolia officinalis*), perilla (*Perilla frutescens*), Saiboku-to, Baikal skullcap (*Scutellaria baicalensis*) or jujube (*Ziziphus vulgaris*).

DiaBeta® (glyburide)   Avoid supplements containing bilberry (*Vaccinium myrtillus*), bitter melon (*Momordica charantia*), ivy gourd (*Coccinia indica*), garlic (*Allium sativum*), ginseng (*Panax ginseng*), gurmar (*Gymnema sylvestre*), onion (*Allium cepa*), Indian kino (*Pterocarpus marsupium*), jambul (*Syzygium cumini*), fenugreek (*Trigonella foenum-graecum*) or salt bush (*Atriplex halimus*).

Diabinese® (chlorpromazine)   Avoid supplements containing bilberry (*Vaccinium myrtillus*), bitter melon (*Momordica charantia*), ivy gourd (*Coccinia indica*), garlic (*Allium sativum*), ginseng (*Panax ginseng*), gurmar (*Gymnema sylvestre*), onion (*Allium cepa*), Indian kino (*Pterocarpus marsupium*), jambul (*Syzygium cumini*), fenugreek (*Trigonella foenum-graecum*) or salt bush (*Atriplex halimus*).

Diazepam (Diastat®, Valium®) Avoid supplements containing kava kava (*Piper methysticum*).

Diclofenac (Arthrotec®, Voltaren®) Avoid supplements containing feverfew (*Tanacetum parthenium*), gossypol (*Gossypium hirsutum*) and white willow (*Salix* species).

Dicyclomine Avoid supplements containing betel nut (*Piper betle*), mandrake (*Mandragora officinarum*) or jimson weed (*Datura stramonium*), a.k.a. thornapple.

Diflunisal (Dolobid®) Avoid supplements containing feverfew (*Tanacetum parthenium*).

Digoxin® Avoid supplements containing ginseng (*Panax ginseng*), eleuthero or Kyushin® (*Eleutherococcus senticosus*), foxglove (*Digitalis purpurea*), false hellebore (*Adonis vernalis*), cascara sagrada *(Rhamnus purshiana),* dogbane (*Apocynum cannabinum*), licorice (*Glycyrrhiza glabra*), plantain (*Plantago lanceolata*), uzara root (*Xysmalobium undulatum*), lily-of-the-valley (*Convallaria majalis*), milkweed (*Apocynum cannabinum*), motherwort (*Leonurus cardiaca*), oleander (*Nerium oleander*), pleurisy root (*Asclepias tuberosa*), senna (*Cassia senna*), St. John's wort (*Hypericum perforatum*), *Strophanthus* species, white squill (*Scilla maritima*), wild ipecac (*Cephaelis ipecacuanha*) or hawthorn (*Crataegus* species).

Dilantin® (phenytoin) Avoid supplements containing evening primrose oil (*Oenothera biennis*), borage oil (*Borago officinalis*) or shankhpushpi (*Convolvulus pluricaulis*).

Diprolene® (betamethasone) Avoid supplements containing licorice (*Glycyrrhiza glabra*), magnolia bark (*Magnolia officinalis*), perilla (*Perilla frutescens*), Saiboku-to, Baikal skullcap (*Scutellaria baicalensis*) or jujube (*Ziziphus vulgaris*).

Dipyridamole (Persantine®) Avoid supplements containing feverfew (*Tanacetum parthenium*), garlic (*Allium sativum*), *Ginkgo biloba* or ginger (*Zingiber officinale*).

Diuril® (chlorthiazide) Avoid supplements containing licorice (*Glycyrrhiza glabra*).

Dolobid® (diflunisal) Avoid supplements containing feverfew (*Tanacetum parthenium*).

Donepezil (Aricept®) Avoid supplements containing betel nut (*Piper betle*), mandrake (*Mandragora officinarum*) or jimson weed (*Datura stramonium*) a.k.a. thornapple.

Doxorubicin (Adriamycin®, Doxil®, Rubex®) Avoid supplements containing 250 mg or more of St. John's wort (*Hypericum perforatum*).

Duraclon® (clonidine HCl) Avoid supplements containing yohimbe (*Pausinystalia yohimbe*).

DynaCirc® (isradipine) Avoid peppermint oil.

Dyrenium® (triamterene) Avoid supplements containing potassium.

Ecotrin® (acetylsalicylic acid) Avoid supplements containing feverfew (*Tanacetum parthenium*).

Edecrin® (ethacrynic acid) Avoid supplements containing licorice (*Glycyrrhiza glabra*), ginseng (*Panax ginseng*), germanium (Ge-Oxy 132) and gossypol (*Gossypium hirsutum*).

Eldepryl® (selegiline) Avoid supplements containing kava kava (*Piper methysticum*).

Enalapril® (ACE inhibitor) Avoid supplements containing 2,000 mg or more of potassium or yohimbe (*Pausinystalia yohimbe*).

Enoxaparin (Lovenox®) Avoid supplements containing feverfew (*Tanacetum parthenium*), garlic (*Allium sativum*), Ginkgo biloba or ginger (*Zingiber officinale*).

Ephredrine Avoid herbs containing salicylates. Avoid herbs high in tannins. (*See listing for aminophylline on page 116 for more details.*) Contraindicated with ma huang or ephedra.

Estradiol (Alora®, Climara®, Estrace®, Estraderm®, Estring®, FemPatch®, Vivelle®) Avoid supplements containing 500 mg or more of ginseng (*Panax ginseng*), *Hoodia* or any human growth hormones.

Estratab® (esterified estrogens) Avoid supplements containing dong quai (*Angelica sinensis*) and ginseng (*Panax ginseng*).

Estratest® (esterified estrogens) Avoid supplements containing dong quai (*Angelica sinensis)* and ginseng (*Panax ginseng*).

Estropipate (Ortho-Est®, Ogen®) Avoid supplements containing ginseng (*Panax ginseng*).

Ethacrynic Acid (Edecrin®) Avoid supplements containing licorice (*Glycyrrhiza glabra*), ginseng (*Panax ginseng*), germanium (Ge-Oxy 132) and gossypol (*Gossypium hirsutum*).

Ethinyl Estradiol Avoid supplements containing ginseng (*Panax ginseng*).

Ethmozine® (moricizine) Avoid supplements containing cascara sagrada (*Rhamnus purshianus*) or licorice (*Glycyrrhiza glabra*).

Etodolac (Lodine®) Avoid supplements containing feverfew (*Tanacetum parthenium*), gossypol (*Gossypium hirsutum*) and white willow (*Salix* species).

Etoposide (VePesid®) Avoid supplements containing St. John's wort (*Hypericum perforatum*).

Etrafon® (perphenazine, amitriptyline) Avoid supplements containing evening primrose oil (*Oenothera biennis*).

Feldene® (piroxicam) Avoid supplements containing feverfew (*Tanacetum parthenium*).

FemPatch® (estradiol) Avoid supplements containing ginseng (*Panax ginseng*).

Fenoprofen (Nalfon®) Avoid supplements containing feverfew (*Tanacetum parthenium*), gossypol (*Gossypium hirsutum*) or white willow (*Salix* species).

Flecainide (Tambocor®) Avoid supplements containing licorice (*Glycyrrhiza glabra*) or cascara sagrada (*Rhamnus purshianus*).

Fluoxetine (Prozac®) Avoid supplements containing St. John's wort (*Hypericum perforatum*) or ayahuasca (*Banisteriopsis caapi*).

Fluphenazine Avoid supplements containing kava kava (*Piper methysticum*) or chasteberry (*Vitex agnus-castus*).

Flurbiprofen Avoid supplements containing feverfew (*Tanacetum parthenium*), gossypol (*Gossypium hirsutum*) or white willow (*Salix* species).

Fluvoxamine (Luvox®) Avoid supplements containing St. John's wort (*Hypericum perforatum*) or ayahuasca (*Banisteriopsis caapi*).

Fragmin® (dalteparin) Avoid supplements containing feverfew (*Tanacetum parthenium*), garlic (*Allium sativum*), *Ginkgo biloba* or ginger (*Zingiber officinale*).

Furosemide (Lasix®) Avoid supplements containing licorice (*Glycyrrhiza glabra*), ginseng (*Panax ginseng*), germanium (Ge-Oxy 132) or gossypol (*Gossypium hirsutum*).

Gabapentin (Neurontin®) Avoid supplements containing *Ginkgo biloba*.

Gen-XENE® (clorazepate) Avoid supplements containing kava kava (*Piper methysticum*).

Glipizide (Glucotrol®) Avoid supplements containing bilberry (*Vaccinium myrtillus*), bitter melon (*Momordica charantia*), ivy gourd (*Coccinia indica*), garlic (*Allium sativum*), ginseng (*Panax ginseng*), gurmar (*Gymnema sylvestre*), onion (*Allium cepa*), Indian kino (*Pterocarpus marsupium*), jambul (*Syzygium cumini*), fenugreek (*Trigonella foenum-graecum*) or salt bush (*Atriplex halimus*).

Glyburide (DiaBeta®, Glynase®, Micronase®) Avoid supplements containing bilberry (*Vaccinium myrtillus*), bitter melon (*Momordica charantia*), ivy gourd (*Coccinia indica*), garlic (*Allium sativum*), ginseng (*Panax ginseng*), gurmar (*Gymnema sylvestre*), onion (*Allium cepa*), Indian kino (*Pterocarpus marsupium*), jambul (*Syzygium cumini*), fenugreek (*Trigonella foenum-graecum*) or salt bush (*Atriplex halimus*).

Halcion® (triazolam) Avoid supplements containing kava kava (*Piper methysticum*).

Haloperidol (Haldol®) Avoid supplements containing kava kava (*Piper methysticum*).

Heparin Avoid supplements containing vitamin K, coenzyme Q10, vitamin D, vitamin E, vitamin C, bromelain, danshen (*Salvia miltiorrhiza*), garlic (*Allium sativum*), ginger (*Zingiber officinale*), goldenseal root (*Hydrastis canadensis*), dong quai root (*Angelica sinensis*), feverfew (*Tanacetum parthenium*) or *Ginkgo biloba*.

Hydralazine   Avoid supplements contaning ephedra (*Ephedra sinica*), yohimbe (*Pausinystalia yohimbe*) or broad bean (*Vicia faba*).

Hydrocortisone Avoid supplements containing licorice (*Glycyrrhiza glabra*), magnolia bark (*Magnolia officinalis*), perilla (*Perilla frutescens*), Saiboku-to, Baikal skullcap (*Scutellaria baicalensis*) or jujube (*Zizyphus vulgaris*).

Hydrodiuril® (hydrochlorthiazide) Avoid supplements containing licorice (*Glycyrrhiza glabra*) or gossypol (*Gossypium hirsutum*).

Ibuprofen Avoid supplements containing white willow (*Salix* species) or feverfew (*Tanacetum parthenium*).

Imipramine Avoid supplements containing St. John's wort (*Hypericum perforatum*).

Imuran® (azathioprine)   Avoid supplements containing andrographis (*Andrographis paniculata*), ashwagandha *(Withania somnifera), Astragalus* species, *Echinacea* species, garlic (*Allium sativum*), ginseng (*Panax ginseng*), maitake (*Grifola frondosa*), reishi (*Ganoderma lucidum*), magnolia vine (*Schisandra chinensis*) or suma (*Pfaffia paniculata*).

Indinavir (Crixivan®)   Avoid supplements containing St. John's wort (*Hypericum perforatum*).

Indocin® (indomethacin)   Avoid supplements containing potassium, gossypol (*Gossypium hirsutum*), white willow (*Salix* species) or feverfew (*Tanacetum parthenium*).

Insulin Avoid supplements containing bilberry (*Vaccinium myrtillus*), bitter melon (*Momordica charantia*), ivy gourd (*Coccinia indica*), garlic (*Allium sativum*), ginseng (*Panax ginseng*), gurmar (*Gymnema sylvestre*), onion (*Allium cepa*), Indian kino (*Pterocarpus marsupium*), jambul (*Syzygium cumini*), fenugreek (*Trigonella foenum-graecum*) or salt bush (*Atriplex halimus*).

Interferon Avoid supplements containing bupleurum (*Bupleurum scorzoneraefolium*).

Ipratropium (Atrovent®, Combivent®)   Avoid supplements containing betel nut (*Piper betle*), mandrake (*Mandragora officinarum*) or jimson weed (*Datura stramonium*) a.k.a. thornapple.

Isoptin® (verapamil) Avoid supplements containing calcium.

Isotretinoin (Amnesteem®, formerly known as Accutane®) Avoid supplements containing more than 25,000 IU of vitamin A.

Isradipine (DynaCirc®) Avoid peppermint oil.

Ketoconazole (Nizoral®) Avoid supplements containing chaparral (*Larrea tridentata*) or *Echinacea* species.

Ketoprofin (Orudis®, Oruvail®) Avoid supplements containing gossypol (*Gossypium hirsutum*), white willow (*Salix* species) or feverfew (*Tanacetum parthenium*).

Ketorolac (Acular®, Toradol®) Avoid supplements containing gossypol (*Gossypium hirsutum*), one gram or more of white willow (*Salix* species) or feverfew (*Tanacetum parthenium*).

Lanoxicaps®, Lanoxin® (digoxin) Avoid supplements containing ginseng (*Panax ginseng*), eleuthero or Kyushin® (*Eleutherococcus senticosus*), foxglove (*Digitalis purpurea*), false hellebore (*Adonis vernalis*), cascara sagrada (*Rhamnus purshianus*), dogbane (*Apocynum cannabinum*), licorice (*Glycyrrhiza glabra*), plantain (*Plantago lanceolata*), uzara root (*Xysmalobium undulatum*), lily-of-the-valley (*Convallaria majalis*), milkweed (*Apocynum cannabinum*), motherwort (*Leonurus cardiaca*), oleander (*Nerium oleander*), pleurisy root (*Asclepias tuberosa*), senna (*Cassia senna*), St. John's wort (*Hypericum perforatum*), *Strophanthus* species, white squill (*Scilla maritima*), wild ipecac (*Cephaelis ipecacuanha*) or hawthorn (*Crataegus* species).

Lansoprazole (Prevacid®) Avoid supplements containing St. John's wort (*Hypericum perforatum*).

Lasix® (furosemide) Avoid supplements containing licorice (*Glycyrrhiza glabra*), ginseng (*Panax ginseng*), geranium (*Ge-Oxy 132*) or gossypol (*Gossypium hirsutum*).

L-Dopa® (levodopa) Avoid supplements containing chasteberry (*Vitex agnus-castus*), kava kava (*Piper methysticum*), large amounts of vitamin B_6 or iron.

Lepirudin (Refludan®) Avoid supplements containing feverfew (*Tanacetum parthenium*), garlic (*Allium sativum*), *Ginkgo biloba* or ginger (*Zingiber officinale*).

Levothyroxine (Synthroid®) Avoid supplements containing iron or kelp (*Fucus vesiculosus*).

Librium® (chlordiazepoxide) Avoid supplements containing kava kava (*Piper methysticum*).

Lodine® (etodolac) Avoid supplements containing feverfew (*Tanacetum parthenium*), gossypol (*Gossypium hirsutum*) and white willow (*Salix* species).

Lorazepam (Ativan®) Avoid supplements containing kava kava (*Piper methysticum*).

Lotrisone® (betamethasone) Avoid supplements containing licorice (*Glycyrrhiza glabra*), magnolia bark (*Magnolia officinalis*), perilla (*Perilla frutescens*), Saiboku-to, Baikal skullcap (*Scutellaria baicalensis*) or jujube (*Ziziphus vulgaris*).

Loxapine (Loxitane®) Avoid supplements containing chasteberry (*Vitex agnus-castus*) or kava kava (*Piper methysticum*).

Lovastatin (Mevacor®) Avoid supplements containing highly soluble fiber.

Lovenox® (enoxaparin) Avoid supplements containing feverfew (*Tanacetum parthenium*), garlic (*Allium sativum*), Ginkgo biloba or ginger (*Zingiber officinale*).

Luvox® (fluvoxamine) Avoid supplements containing St. John's wort (*Hypericum perforatum*) or ayahuasca (*Banisteriopsis caapi*).

Mebaral® (mephobarbital) Avoid supplements containing valerian (*Valeriana officinalis*), evening primrose oil (*Oenothera biennis*), borage oil (*Borago officinalis*) or kava kava (*Piper methysticum*).

Methimazole (Tapazole®) Avoid supplements containing kelp (*Fucus vesiculosus*).

Methotrexate Avoid supplements containing *Echinacea* species.

Methyldopa (Aldomet®) Avoid supplements containing 10 mg or more of iron.

Mevacor® (Lovastatin) Avoid supplements containing highly soluble fiber.

Micronase® (glyburide) Avoid supplements containing bilberry (*Vaccinium myrtillus*), bitter melon (*Momordica charantia*), ivy gourd (*Coccinia indica*), garlic (*Allium sativum*), ginseng (*Panax ginseng*), gurmar (*Gymnema sylvestre*), onion (*Allium cepa*), Indian kino (*Pterocarpus marsupium*), jambul (*Syzygium cumini*), fenugreek (*Trigonella foenum-graecum*) or salt bush (*Atriplex halimus*).

Midamor® (amiloride HCl) Avoid supplements containing potassium or 500 mg or more of licorice (*Glycyrrhiza glabra*).

Moduretic® (amiloride HCl) Avoid supplements containing potassium or 500 mg or more of licorice (*Glycyrrhiza glabra*).

Moricizine (Ethmozine®) Avoid supplements containing cascara sagrada (*Rhamnus purshianus*) or licorice (*Glycyrrhiza glabra*).

Motrin® (ibuprofen) Avoid supplements containing white willow (*Salix* species) or feverfew (*Tanacetum parthenium*).

Nalfon® (fenoprofen) Avoid supplements containing feverfew (*Tanacetum parthenium*), gossypol (*Gossypium hirsutum*) or white willow (*Salix* species).

Nardil® (phenelzine) Avoid supplements containing St. John's wort (*Hypericum perforatum*), ginseng (*Panax ginseng*), cayenne pepper (*Capsicum annuum*) or Scotch broom (*Cytisus scoparius*).

Naproxen (Anaprox®) Avoid supplements containing feverfew (*Tanacetum parthenium*).

Nembutal® (pentobarbital) Avoid supplements containing valerian (*Valeriana officinalis*), evening primrose oil (*Oenothera biennis*), borage oil (*Borago officinalis*) or kava kava (*Piper methysticum*).

NeoDecadron® (dexamethasone) Avoid supplements containing licorice (*Glycyrrhiza glabra*), magnolia bark (*Magnolia officinalis*), perilla (*Perilla frutescens),* Saiboku-to, Baikal skullcap (*Scutellaria baicalensis*) or jujube (*Ziziphus vulgaris).*

Neoral® (cyclosporine) Avoid supplements containing *Echinacea* species and St. John's wort (*Hypericum perforatum*).

Neurontin® (gabapentin) Avoid supplements containing *Ginkgo biloba*.

Nizoral® (ketoconazole) Avoid supplements containing chaparral (*Larrea tridentata*), or *Echinacea* species.

Normiflo® (ardeparin sodium) Avoid supplements containing feverfew (*Tanacetum parthenium*), garlic (*Allium sativum*), *Ginkgo biloba* or ginger (*Zingiber officinale*).

Ogen® (estropipate) Avoid supplements containing ginseng (*Panax ginseng*).

Orgaran® (danaparoid) Avoid supplements containing feverfew (*Tanacetum parthenium*), garlic (*Allium sativum*), ginkgo (*Ginkgo biloba*) or ginger (*Zingiber officinale*).

Ortho-Est® (estropipate) Avoid supplements containing ginseng (*Panax ginseng*).

Orudis®, Oruvail® (Ketoprofin) Avoid supplements containing gossypol (*Gossypium hirsutum*), white willow (*Salix* species) or feverfew (*Tanacetum parthenium*).

Oxaprozin (Daypro®) Avoid supplements containing feverfew (*Tanacetum parthenium*).

Pacerone® (amiodarone) Avoid supplements containing *Echinacea* species, licorice (*Glycyrrhiza glabra*) or cascara sagrada (*Rhamnus purshianus*).

Parlodel® (bromocriptine) Avoid supplements containing chasteberry (*Vitex agnus-castus*).

Parnate® (tranylcypromine) Avoid supplements containing St. John's wort (*Hypericum perforatum*), ginseng (*Panax ginseng*), cayenne pepper (*Capsicum annuum*) or Scotch broom (*Cytisus scoparius*).

Penicillamine (Cuprimine®, Depen®) Avoid supplements containing copper or iron.

Pentobarbital (Nembutal®) Avoid supplements containing valerian (*Valeriana officinalis*), evening primrose oil (*Oenothera biennis*), borage oil (*Borago officinalis*) or kava kava (*Piper methysticum*).

Phenelzine (Nardil®) Avoid supplements containing St. John's wort (*Hypericum perforatum*), ginseng (*Panax ginseng*), cayenne pepper (*Capsicum annuum*) or Scotch broom (*Cytisus scoparius*).

Phenytoin (Dilantin®)   Avoid supplements containing evening primrose oil (*Oenothera biennis*), borage oil (*Borago officinalis*) and shankhpushpi (*Convolvulus pluricaulis*).

Piroxicam (Feldene®)   Avoid supplements containing feverfew (*Tanacetum parthenium*).

Plavix® (clopidogrel)   Avoid supplements containing feverfew (*Tanacetum parthenium*), garlic (*Allium sativum*), *Ginkgo biloba* or ginger (*Zingiber officinale*).

Pravachol® (pravastatin)   Avoid supplements containing highly soluble fiber.

Prevacid® (lansoprazole)   Avoid supplements containing St. John's wort (*Hypericum perforatum*).

Prochlorperazine (Compazine®)   Avoid supplements containing evening primrose oil (*Oenothera biennis*).

Prozac® (fluoxetine)   Avoid supplements containing St. John's wort (*Hypericum perforatum*) or ayahuasca (*Banisteriopsis caapi*).

Pseudoephedrine   Avoid herbs containing salicylates. Avoid herbs high in tannins. (*See listing for aminophylline on page 116 for more details.*) Contraindicated with ma huang or ephedra.

Questran® (cholestyramine)   May bind to herbal supplements, thereby preventing absorption.

Refludan® (lepirudin)   Avoid supplements containing feverfew (*Tanacetum parthenium*), garlic (*Allium sativum*), *Ginkgo biloba* or ginger (*Zingiber officinale*).

Reopro® (Abciximab)   Avoid supplements containing feverfew (*Tanacetum parthenium*), garlic (*Allium sativum*), *Ginkgo biloba* or ginger (*Zingiber officinale*).

Rubex® (doxorubicin)   Avoid supplements containing more than 250 mg of St. John's wort (*Hypericum perforatum*).

Sandimmune® (cyclosporine)   Avoid supplements containing *Echinacea* species and St. John's wort (*Hypericum perforatum*).

Selegiline (Eldepryl®) Avoid supplements containing kava kava (*Piper methysticum*).

Septra® (sulfamethoxazole, trimethoprim) Avoid supplements containing potassium.

Simulect® (basiliximab) Avoid supplements containing andrographis (*Andrographis paniculata*), ashwagandha *(Withania somnifera)*, *Astragalus* species, *Echinacea* species, garlic (*Allium sativum*), ginseng (*Panax ginseng*), maitake (*Grifola frondosa*), reishi (*Ganoderma lucidum*), magnolia vine (*Schisandra chinensis*) or suma (*Pfaffia paniculata*).

Sinemet® (carbidopa) Avoid supplements containing iron or kava kava (*Piper methysticum*).

Sotalol (Betapace®) Avoid supplements containing licorice (*Glycyrrhiza glabra*) or cascara sagrada (*Rhamnus purshianus*).

Spironolactone (Aldactone®) Avoid supplements containing large amounts of potassium (2,000 mg or more) or licorice (*Glycyrrhiza glabra*).

Sucralfate (Carafate®) May bind to herbal supplements, thereby preventing absorption.

Sulindac (Clinoril®) Avoid supplements containing feverfew (*Tanacetum parthenium*).

Symmetrel® (Amantadine HCI) Avoid supplements containing 250 mg or more of chasteberry (*Vitex agnus-castus*) or Oregon grape (*Mahonia aquifolium*).

Synthroid® (levothyroxine) Avoid supplements containing iron or kelp (*Fucus vesiculosus*).

Tambocor® (flecainide) Avoid supplements containing licorice (*Glycyrrhiza glabra*) or cascara sagrada (*Rhamnus purshianus*).

Tapazole® (methimazole) Avoid supplements containing kelp (*Fucus vesiculosus*).

Tetracycline When using tetracycline to treat cholera, avoid supplements containing goldenseal (*Hydrastis canadensis*), barberry (*Berberis vulgaris*) or Oregon grape (*Mahonia aquifolium*).

Theophylline (Aminophylline®) Salicylates interfere with absorption when taken simultaneously. Thus, avoid meadowsweet herb (*Filipendula ulmaria*), poplar herb (*Populus* species), 500 mg or more of willow bark (*Salix* species) or wintergreen (*Gaultheria procumbens, Pyrola rotundifolia*). Herbs high in tannins also impair absorption if taken simultaneously so avoid green or black tea (*Camellia sinensis*), uva ursi (*Arctostaphylos uva-ursi*), black walnut (*Juglans nigra*), red raspberry (*Rubus idaeus*), oak (*Quercus robur*) or witch hazel (*Hamamelis virginiana*).

Thorazine® (chlorpromazine) Avoid supplements containing chasteberry (*Vitex agnus-castus*) or kava kava (*Piper methysticum*).

TobraDex® (dexamethasone) Avoid supplements containing licorice (*Glycyrrhiza glabra*), magnolia bark (*Magnolia officinalis*), perilla (*Perilla frutescens*), Saiboku-to, Baikal skullcap (*Scutellaria baicalensis*) or jujube (*Ziziphus vulgaris*).

Toradol® (Ketorolac) Avoid supplements containing gossypol (*Gossypium hirsutum*), white willow (*Salix* species) or feverfew (*Tanacetum parthenium*).

Tranxene® (clorazepate) Avoid supplements containing kava kava (*Piper methysticum*).

Tranylcypromine (Parnate®) Avoid supplements containing St. John's wort (*Hypericum perforatum*), ginseng (*Panax ginseng*), cayenne pepper (*Capsicum annuum*) or Scotch broom (*Cytisus scoparius*).

Triamterene (Dyrenium®) Avoid supplements containing potassium.

Triazolam (Halcion®) Avoid supplements containing kava kava (*Piper methysticum*).

Urecholine® (bethanechol) Avoid supplements containing betel nut (*Piper betle*), mandrake (*Mandragora officinarum*) or jimson weed (*Datura stramonium*) a.k.a. thornapple.

Valium® (diazepam) Avoid supplements containing kava kava (*Piper methysticum*).

VePesid® (Etoposide) Avoid supplements containing St. John's wort (*Hypericum perforatum*).

Verapamil (Verelan®, Calan®) Avoid supplements containing calcium, licorice (*Glycyrrhiza glabra*) and cascara sagrada (*Rhamnus purshianus*).

Verelan® (verapamil) Avoid supplements containing calcium, licorice (*Glycyrrhiza glabra*) and cascara sagrada (*Rhamnus purshianus).*

Vivelle® (estradiol) Avoid supplements containing *Panax ginseng.*

Voltaren® (diclofenac) Avoid supplements containing feverfew (*Tanacetum parthenium*), gossypol (*Gossypium hirsutum)* and white willow (*Salix* species).

Warfarin (Coumadin®) Avoid supplements containing vitamin K, coenzyme Q10, vitamin D, vitamin E, vitamin C, bromelain, danshen (*Salvia miltiorrhiza*), garlic (*Allium sativum*), feverfew (*Tanacetum parthenium*), ginseng (*Panax ginseng*), ginger (*Zingiber officinale*), dong quai root, (*Angelica sinensis*), *Ginkgo biloba* or vinpocetine.

Xanax® (alprazolam) Avoid supplements containing kava kava (*Piper methysticum*), false unicorn (*Chamaelirium luteum*) or chamomile.

Zenapax® (daclizumab) Avoid supplements containing andrographis (*Andrographis paniculata*), ashwagandha (*Withania somnifera),* *Astragalus* species, *Echinacea species*, garlic (*Allium sativum*), ginseng (*Panax ginseng*), maitake (*Grifola frondosa*), reishi (*Ganoderma lucidum*), magnolia vine (*Schisandra chinensis*) or suma (*Pfaffia paniculata*).

The Future

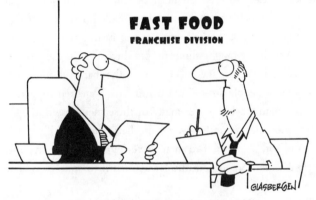

FAST FOOD
FRANCHISE DIVISION

"Our challenge is to convince the public that heart attacks are sexy."

From the turn of the 20th century to the mid-1990s, many famous herbalists who were against FDA intervention in health-care were forced to work and teach covertly, or "underground." Many who chose not to go underground faced being jailed for "dispensing herbs for the purpose of healing" without a proper license. Among the great healers and teachers of the 20th century are Samuel Thompson, founder of Thompsonian Medicine; Jethro Kloss, author of *Back to Eden*; Gaston Naessens, inventor of the dark field microscope, which makes it easier to examine live biological samples; Dr. Bernard Jensen, founder of modern iridology; and John R. Christopher, the first person to encapsulate herbs.

These men and others were sometimes pursued and taken to court for healing and helping people with natural foods and herbs. They suffered many hardships including trials, imprisonment, death threats, financial devastation and ridicule, all because they believed that herbs were made for the use of man and that patenting herbal remedies was a sin against God and humanity. They taught about proper diets, regular exercise and the avoidance of caffeine, nicotine and other harmful substances. Millions of people around the world have benefited from their writings and teachings, yet many of these men passed away in poverty or spent months away from their families while on trial or in prison. We owe it to their posterity to recognize them for their endurance and commitment to truth in spite of ridicule and shame.

Now, more than a decade after the turn of a new millennium, herbology has not changed. What has been changing is the way science is looking at herbal medicine. Through many modern diagnostic tools, the allopathic community is beginning to recognize and document the benefits of herbs and the phytochemicals that make them beneficial. Unfortunately, this recognition seems to be motivated not by goodwill but instead by greed. The herbal industry's profits are growing yearly, and many pharmaceutical companies are missing out on the profits.

The future for the herbal medicine industry is a forked road. On one hand, through education and self-regulation, many new and beneficial uses for plants could be discovered and integrated into allopathic communities. Hospitals and research institutions across the country have already documented a good deal of success using "alternative" treatments of degenerative diseases. These include color therapy, a technique that uses color and light to balance the body; hydrotherapy, which incorporates water for pain relief and disease healing; biofeedback, a technique that helps patients learn to control involuntary bodily reactions such as heart rate and muscle tension; acupuncture, which uses needles inserted in various points of the body to relieve pain; and other traditional modalities used in conjunction with herbs and/or allopathic treatments.

The other fork in this road to the future could possibly lead to the total destruction of herbal traditions. As pharmaceutical companies lobby the federal government to regulate herbs in order to capture the market and turn profits toward themselves, we may see increasing government regulations and oversight of the herbal medicine industry.

We had a glimpse of the possible ramifications of government intervention with the trial of the case against the herb ma huang (ephedra), which contains the phytochemical ephedrine. For years this herb has been used as a safe alternative treatment for bronchitis and asthma. However, in the late 1990s, Metabolife® International included ephedra in their popular diet product Metabolife®. Of its hundreds of thousands of users, there were a number of adverse events implicated with the use of this product. After a lengthy trial period, which cost taxpayers millions of dollars, the FDA banned dietary supplements containing ephedra in 2004.

All foods contain phytochemicals, which have medicinal uses and should be used with wisdom and moderation. We can't expect the government to regulate this industry for us. If they did, there would be a warning label on every fruit and vegetable in the produce section. If we continue to follow this fork, a new medical "dark age" will occur as natural cures to common ailments and degenerative diseases are kept from the public. A sick population is naturally more profitable to pharmaceutical companies. Institutes such as the American Cancer Association, AIDS Research Foundation and American Diabetes Association receive billions of dollars of federal and corporate funding to fight these diseases, yet the cures have yet to be discovered. Much of the funding has been spent on early diagnostic technology, which is set up so you can now be diagnosed earlier and take a drug sooner, further stuffing the pockets of the drug companies.

Which fork we will take is up to the people—it's up to you! As long as the United States remains a democratic republic, the people still control which direction we take. Though capitalism drives this country, it cannot overrule individual rights unless the people allow it to do so.

A wellness renaissance must occur, and it is the people who must initiate it. If we let insurance companies decide which treatments they will cover and which they will not, where is our freedom of choice? If we allow the government to decide what foods we can and can't eat and what drugs we can and can't take, then we have lost our freedom to govern ourselves. You can and should have the power to decide which treatments to use for yourself and your loved ones. Knowledge is the key to making an informed decision. The drug companies, the government and insurance companies do not believe that you have the capability to gain the knowledge necessary to make that choice for yourself. This book will prove them wrong. Put to use the knowledge found here. Seek out other good books as well. Question the system and question the information in the different books you read. It is your right and your duty as the primary caregiver of yourself and your family to question. If we do not empower ourselves and govern ourselves, then the government or insurance companies will do it for us. Which do you prefer?

Appendix A: Growing Selected Home Pharmacy Herbs

Aloe Vera

Aloe vera is one of several aloe varieties, so make sure you plant aloe *vera*. Since aloe vera is native to deserts, it grows well with fast-draining sandy soil, lots of sunlight and little water. Buy a starter plant from a garden shop. As the plant matures and smaller plants start to grow around its base, remove and replant those buds to start new plants.

Keep aloe vera plants indoors except in very warm climates (where temperatures generally stay above 30 degrees Fahrenheit), and allow them to dry completely between thorough waterings. Aloe vera's roots spread out horizontally rather than vertically, so when repotting plants that have outgrown their containers, choose a pot that is wide instead of deep. Choose one that drains quickly. Use well-fertilized soil or cacti potting mix to make sure the aloe vera receives adequate nutrients.

To harvest part of the aloe vera plant, cut off one of the outer leaves close to the base so that the plant can continue growing from the center.

Cayenne Pepper

Cayenne pepper can be grown from seeds, but it's easier to buy plants from a garden center. Choose plants that do not have flowers or fruit on them. If you choose to start with seeds, plant them in very shallow, lightweight soil and keep them moist but not wet. Pepper plants grow better in warm conditions, so keep the seedlings in a sunny spot in the house or in a greenhouse. Seeds should start to sprout in two to three weeks. After a month, the plants should be replanted in moist, fertilized soil.

Cayenne plants can grow up to four feet tall and two feet wide and should therefore be given plenty of room. Space the plants 18 to 24 inches apart in a well-drained place where they will have full sunshine and minimal shade, except during the hottest part of the day, when they may get scorched. Keep the soil moist but not soggy.

Peppers are ready to pick approximately three months after planting, when the peppers are about four to six inches long, firm to the touch and remove easily from the plant when tugged gently.

Cinnamon

Growing cinnamon is a little different from growing the rest of the herbs in this section, since cinnamon comes from trees that can grow up to 50 feet tall. Cinnamon needs to be planted in a very warm climate—cinnamon trees are native to areas with hot and humid climates like Sri Lanka, Vietnam and Bangladesh. More tropical climates where temperatures do not usually fall below 20 degrees Fahrenheit are the only ones were growing cinnamon trees is feasible.

Although you don't have to wait for your plant to grow into a 50-foot tree before you can harvest cinnamon, you will need a lot of space and a lot of patience: a tree will be between two and eight years old before you can harvest the bark from the shoots and dry the inner bark to make cinnamon sticks. There are several species of cinnamon. The variety generally preferred in the United States is *Cinnamomum aromaticum*, which has a stronger flavor than *C. verum*, or "true cinnamon." Research the particular type of cinnamon tree you're cultivating to make sure you know when to harvest it.

Plant cinnamon seeds 1/2 inch deep in warm, moist, rich, well-drained soil in partially shaded sunlight. The best time to plant is in the spring, when plants will have the most time possible to grow before the next bout of colder weather arrives.

Keep the soil around the tree moist, but make sure it's not soggy. Fertilize the soil every month until the seedlings are well established, and protect the tree from hard frosts. After growing for three years, the tree will need to be pruned every other year to encourage the roots to send up shoots, which are the part of the tree you'll be harvesting.

To harvest the cinnamon, allow shoots to grow for one year before removing the bark and then peeling out the inner bark in strips. Allow the strips of inner bark to dry and you will have cinnamon sticks for use in your next herbal remedy.

Dandelion

The easiest way to cultivate dandelion roots is to simply allow the hearty weeds to grow in your lawn. Letting them thrive is easier than trying to eliminate them! If you prefer to keep such weeds separate from your lawn, purchase seeds and plant them somewhere separate from the rest of your lawn. Planting dandelions away from the lawn also makes it easier to harvest the roots.

Finding dandelion seeds to purchase may be tricky, but dandelion greens are considered quite a delicacy in Europe, so try online vendors if a garden store doesn't carry the seeds.

Dandelions grow without much help. But to ensure productive plants, plant them about six inches apart in rich soil and keep them moist. To harvest the roots later, consider planting seeds in planters rather than in a garden bed. Dandelion roots grow straight down and can be 18 inches long or longer, so trying to extract them from a regular garden is much more difficult than pulling them from a 12-inch-deep pot.

When the plants are three months old, they're ready to harvest. Pulling on dandelion plants generally leaves you with a stalk in your hand while the roots stay firmly in the ground. Avoid this by thoroughly wetting the soil before attempting a harvest. When dandelions aren't growing in the middle of a lawn, the roots aren't tangled with other plants and should be much easier to pull. Dry the roots in the sun and use them in your home pharmacy recipes.

Echinacea Roots

The echinacea plant produces beautiful flowers in the summer, so you'll be able to enjoy it long before the roots reach harvestable maturity, which takes three years. You can probably buy echinacea plants at your local garden center, but it's better to start from seeds to make sure the plants are as healthy as possible.

Like most plants, echinacea grows best in rich, well-drained soil and good sunshine. Plant them about 1/4 inch deep and two to four inches apart in an area that gets full sunshine. The seeds need a little cold weather while germinating, so planting them in the early fall or early spring is a good idea.

The seeds should sprout in two or three weeks, and you'll need to thin them so they are at least six inches apart. Larger varieties of echinacea will need even more room. *Echinacea purpurea*, for example, grows so large you'll want to make sure individual plants are at least 18 inches apart.

Echinacea can stand cold weather, but it does much better in fairly dry, well-drained soil than it does in wet or soggy soil. Light watering is sufficient.

Echinacea roots will be ready to harvest after three years. Wait until the plants have weathered several hard frosts, and harvest the roots during the plant's dormant period, usually in late autumn, when the plant has dried and the flowers have gone to seed. Dig up the entire plant and cut off the portions of root you want to harvest, then replant the remainder of the plant. Wash the harvested roots thoroughly and allow them to dry completely before using them.

Garlic

Garlic plants need loose, nutrient-rich soil, plenty of sun and a little water. There is no need to purchase a special garlic seed— just plant a few cloves. Each clove will grow into a plant with a new bulb, and each bulb will have several cloves, making a garlic crop self-sustaining.

Garlic cloves are activated for growing by cold temperatures, so it's common to plant them in the late fall or early winter, generally after the first frost. If you live in a warmer climate, chill your garlic before planting it. Refrigerating it for six to eight weeks does the trick.

Garlic shoots, the signs of the plant, should appear in the early spring for garlic planted in cold climates in late October or early November. Shoots will emerge much sooner in warmer climates because it does not lie dormant during the cold months.

Plant individual cloves, not an entire garlic bulb. Before planting, prepare the soil with fertilizer or compost and make sure it is loose enough for a garlic bulb to grow nice and plump without any restrictions. Planting large cloves yields large bulbs; smaller cloves will produce smaller bulbs.

Before planting, split the papery skin of the garlic and separate the cloves. Plant individual cloves pointed side up, one to two inches deep and four to six inches apart. Since garlic needs good soil and needs to be well drained, plant garlic in raised beds or deep containers so the nutrients don't get depleted too quickly and the bulbs are kept out of standing water. Keep the plants in a cool location where they'll get plenty of sun, and keep them damp but not wet.

Garlic is ready to harvest when the leaves are almost entirely brown. Dig it up—don't pull, or the leaves will pull off, leaving the bulb in the soil. Rinse off the dirt, and then hang the bulbs to dry.

Ginger

Ginger root may be purchased at most grocery stores. But to take your home pharmacy to the next level, cultivate your own plant. To start, use a root from grocery store. To make sure the root is as fresh as possible, look for one about four to five inches long that is plump (rather than withered) and that has green color on the ends of its "fingers." If you can't find one that appears greenish, pick the freshest-looking root and you should be able to grow a healthy plant.

Plant just a couple of pieces of the root. Cut or break off 1- or 2-inch long sections, making sure that each one has one or two buds (little bumps) on it. Let the sections dry for 24–48 hours, then plant them 12 inches apart and no more than one inch deep in rich, loose soil. Ginger plants thrive in shade, so plant them out of direct sunlight. Remember, it's the root you're cultivating, so make sure each root section has plenty of soft, nutrient-rich soil around it so it can grow a big, healthy root.

Once you've planted the ginger, water it thoroughly and keep it wet until leaves emerge. At that point diminish frequency of watering, but make sure the soil is never completely dry. Thoroughly soak the plant each time you water, typically once a week.

In about 10 months, the root will be ready to harvest. Gently pull the entire plant from the soil. To keep growing ginger, break off a small section of the root that still has a plant attached and replant that for a later harvest. Remove the foliage from the remainder of the root and wash the root. Keep it in the refrigerator to delay shriveling and prolong potency.

Lemongrass

Beginning from an existing plant is the easiest way to start your own crop of lemongrass if the climate of your area is appropriate. Lemongrass only grows in climates where minimum temperatures do not typically fall below −10 degrees Fahrenheit.

Lemongrass can be purchased at many large grocery stores or Asian food stores. Buy the freshest looking plant you can find, preferably one with traces of roots still on the bottom of the stalk, then cut a few inches off the top and peel off any dry, dead-looking outer layers. Put the stalk in a glass with an inch or two of water in it and place it on a windowsill where it will get plenty of sunlight. Roots should start to sprout within a week or two.

Once the roots are about two inches long, the plant is ready for soil. Plant it in rich, well-drained soil so that the base is just below the surface. Keep the plant in a sunny location and water it enough that it is always moist but not soggy. As long as you protect your plant from cold temperatures, it should last all year long. If you live in a warm climate and plant it outside, it could grow to be up to five feet tall and five feet wide.

To harvest lemongrass, simply cut off a few leaves at a time and dry them or use them fresh.

Oregano

To grow oregano, start with seeds or cuttings (small clippings) of an existing plant. Cuttings can be planted immediately, but seeds need to sprout first. To sprout seeds, sprinkle them in a plastic container, mist them with water and cover the container with plastic wrap. Set the container in a place where it will get plenty of sunlight, and you should have sprouts within about a week. Plant the sprouts outdoors in a well-drained area after the last frost, or plant them indoors at any time of year.

Oregano thrives in desert-like conditions, so keep the plants in sunlight. Water when the soil has dried out completely.

Oregano is ready to harvest when the plants are four to six inches tall. Cut the stem down to the last two pairs of leaves.

The plant will soon sprout new leaves, and you will have wonderfully fresh oregano to use in your favorite recipes or herbal remedies. For the most aromatic, flavorful oregano, harvest it just as buds are starting to form, or pinch off the buds so the plant won't expend its energy and nutrients on the flowers—even though oregano flowers are beautiful.

Dry the leaves in a cool, dark, ventilated location or freeze them whole. Either way, store them in an airtight container to maintain potency.

Oregano plants grown indoors can continue to yield new leaves for harvesting all year. Outdoor plants will need to be protected from frost, but they can also be perennials if you cut them down and cover them with mulch before the temperature sinks below freezing.

Peppermint

Peppermint plants can be grown from seeds or cuttings. To use cuttings, simply cut off a piece of an existing plant that has roots attached and replant the new piece. You'll soon have a sturdy new plant. To cultivate peppermint from seeds, plant seeds about 1/3 inch deep and two inches apart in rich, moist soil. Once the seedlings are two to four inches tall, thin or transplant them so they are 12 inches apart. Either cultivation technique requires rich soil, constant moisture, good drainage and plenty of sunshine.

You can begin harvesting the leaves when the plants are about 12 inches tall. Harvest only a few at a time, and pick the larger, outside leaves so the plant has time to replace them.

Rose Hips

Many different varieties of rose bushes produce rose hips, but the most common variety used for this purpose is the rugosa heirloom rose.

To cultivate rose hips, plant and care for a rose bush as you normally would, but do not remove old blossoms when they are spent. Allow them to remain on the bush. After a few weeks, rose hips will start to develop.

Rose hips are ready to harvest when they are a bright reddish orange or red. Orange hips are not yet ripe, and dark red hips are past maturity.

Sage

Sage is a hardy plant that requires full sunlight and well-drained soil. Start seeds in small pots and cover them lightly with rich soil. Keep the soil moist as the seeds are sprouting, which may take up to six weeks, then thin seedlings to about 12 inches apart.

In about another month, the seedlings will be ready for transplanting to larger pots, as each plant can grow up to two feet tall. Larger plants need less water—water them lightly once or twice a week and allow the soil to dry a bit between waterings.

Once your plants are established, they will last for years. Keep them pruned down so they don't get scraggly.

Harvest the leaves as needed, but it's best to wait until the plant is well-established to take more than a few leaves at a time. Remove individual leaves or cut the entire stem to harvest the central leaves. Younger leaves are more tender and flavorful.

Appendix B: Suppliers

NutraNomics:

www.nutranomics.com or toll-free 1-800-745-0393

This company provides all-natural, effective dietary supplements. NutraNomics® products have no fillers, no flow agents, and they do not buy herbs from China. If you do not have time to use the *My Home Pharmacy* recipes at home, try some of the many wonderful products available through NutraNomics®, all of which I formulated.

Grandma's Country Foods:

www.grandmascountryfoods.com

This company is my preferred source for bulk food items, cookware, emergency supplies and many other useful items. Fast, friendly and cost effective.

Mountain Rose Herbs:

www.mountainroseherbs.com or 1-800-879-3337

A very fine supplier for all your home herbal needs from bulk herbs and spices to essential oils, organic beeswax, butters and clays. They provide great prices, excellent customer service and shipping to any country in the world.

San Francisco Herb Company:

www.sfherb.com or 1-800-227-4530

This company is a great and economical supplier of bulk herbs. They will typically sell in smaller quantities so you won't have to store whole buckets of herbs at home.

Aroma Tools:

www.aromatools.com

A source of pure ingestible essential oils, fractionated coconut oils and other essential oil tools.

To contact Tracy Gibbs, please send e-mails to:
tracysherbs@gmail.com

References

Akhondzadeh S., Noroozian M., et al. "*Salvia officinalis* extract in the treatment of patients with mild to moderate Alzheimer's disease: a double blind, randomized and placebo-controlled trial." *Journal of Clinical Pharmacy and Therapeutics* 28, no. 1 (2003): 53–59.

Anderson. R.N. "Deaths: Leading Causes for 2000." *National Vital Statistics Reports* 50, no. 16 (2002).

Ankri, S. and D. Mirelman. "Antimicrobial properties of allicin from garlic." *Microbes and Infection* 1, no. 2 (1999): 125–9.

Apariman, S., S. Ratchanon, et al. "Effectiveness of ginger for prevention of nausea and vomiting after gynecological laparoscopy." *Journal of the Medical Association of Thailand* 89, no. 12 (2006): 2003–09.

Badell, M.L., S.M. Ramin, et al. "Treatment options for nausea and vomiting during pregnancy." *Pharmacology* 26, no. 9 (2006): 1273–87.

Betancur-Galvis, L., et al. "Antitumor and antiviral activity of Colombian medicinal plant extracts." *Memórias do Instituto Oswaldo Cruz* 94, no. 4 (1999): 531–35.

Bortolotti M., G. Coccia, et al. "The treatment of functional dyspepsia with red pepper." *Alimentary Pharmacology and Therapeutics* 16, no. 6 (2002): 1075–82.

Bown, S.R. *Scurvy: How a Surgeon, a Mariner, and a Gentleman Solved the Greatest Medical Mystery of the Age of Sail.* New York: Thomas Dunne Books, 2003.

Carrick, P. "Medical Ethics in the Ancient World." *Clinical Medical Ethics.* Washington, D.C.: Georgetown University Press, 2001.

Chrubasik C., R.K. Duke and S. Chrubasik. "The evidence for clinical efficacy of rose hip and seed: a systematic review." *Phytotherapy Research* 20, no. 1 (2006): 1–3.

Ciabatti P.G., L. D'Ascanio. "Intranasal capsicum spray in idiopathic rhinitis: a randomized prospective application regimen trial." *Acta Oto-Laryngologica* 129, no. 4 (2009): 367–71.

Cutler, R.R. and P. Wilson. "Antibacterial activity of a new, stable, aqueous extract of allicin against methicillan-resistant *Staphylococcus aureus.*" *British Journal of Biomedical Science* 61, no. 2 (2004): 71–74.

Fishbein, M. *Modern Home Medical Advisor.* P.F. Collier & Son, 1976.

Fowler J.F. Jr., H. Woolery-Lloyd, et al. "Innovations in natural ingredients and their use in skin care." *Journal of Drugs in Dermatology* 9, no. 6 (2010): S72–81.

Gagnier J.J., M.W. van Tulder, et al. "Herbal medicine for low back pain: a Cochrane review." *Spine* 32, no. 1 (2007): 82–92.

Hoffman, D. *The Information Source Book of Herbal Medicine.* The Crossing Press, 1994.

Jaramillo, M.C., et al. "Cytotoxicity and antileishmanial activity of *Annona muricata* pericarp." *Fitoterapia* 71, no. 2 (2000): 183–86.

Jefferson, T. *Notes on Virginia* Q.XVII, 1782. ME 2:222.

Jensen, B. *Herbs: Wonder Healers.* Bernard Jensen, 1992.

Khan A., M. Safdar, et al. "Cinnamon improves glucose and lipids of people with type 2 diabetes." *Diabetes Care* 26, no. 12 (2003): 3215–18.

Kloss, J. *Back to Eden.* Woodbridge, 1939.

Langmead, L., R.J. Makins, D.S. Rampton. "Anti-inflammatory effects of aloe vera gel in human colorectal mucosa in vitro." *Alimentary Pharmacology & Therapeutics* 19, no. 5 (2004): 521–27.

López P., C. Sánchez, et al. "Solid- and vapor-phase antimicrobial activities of six essential oils: susceptibility of selected foodborne bacterial and fungal strains." *Journal of Agriculture and Food Chemistry* 53, no. 17 (2005): 6939–46.

Lust, J. *The Herb Book.* Benedict Lust, 1974.

Ma Y.X., Y. Zhu, et al. "The aging retarding effect of 'Long-Life CiLi'." *Mechanisms of Ageing and Development* 96, no. 1–3 (1997): 171–80.

Mansell, P.W., H. Ichinose, et al. "Macrophage destruction of human malignant cells in vivo." *Journal of the National Cancer Institute* 54, no. 3 (1975): 571–80.

Masood, N., A. Chaudhry, et al. "Antibacterial effects of oregano (*Origanum vulgare*) against gram negative bacilli." *Pakistan Journal of Botany* 39, no. 2 (2007): 609–13.

Merck Manual. 16th ed. Merck Research Laboratories, 1992.

Myers, S. "Facing Biological Degeneration." HSR Science Series. HSR Press, 2004.

O'Hara M., D. Kiefer, et al. "A Review of 12 Commonly Used Medicinal Herbs." *Archives of Family Medicine* 7, no. 7 (1998): 523–36.

Ozdemir B., A. Ekbul, et al. "Effects of *Origanum onites* on endothelial function and serum biochemical markers in hyperlipidaemic patients." *Journal of International Medical Research* 36, no. 6 (2008): 1326–34.

Pozzatti, P., L.A. Scheid, et al. "In vitro activity of essential oils extracted from plants used as spices against fluconazole-resistant and fluconazole-susceptible *Candida* spp." *Canadian Journal of Microbiology* 54, no. 11 (2008): 950–56.

Reinhart K.M., C.I. Coleman, et al. "Effects of garlic on blood pressure in patients with and without systolic hypertension: a meta-analysis." *The Annals of Pharmacotherapy* 42 no. 12 (2008): 1766–71.

Richardson, J. *Health and Longevity.* Home Health Society, 1910.

Santillo, H. *Natural Healing with Herbs.* Hohm, 1984.

Shah, S.A., S. Sander, et al. "Evaluation of echinacea for the prevention and treatment of the common cold: a meta-analysis." *The Lancet Infectious Diseases* 7, no. 7 (2007): 473–80.

Sheng Y. "Induction of apoptosis and inhibition of proliferation in human tumor cells treated with extracts of Uncaria tomentosa." *Anticancer Research* 18, no. 5A (1998): 3363–68.

Shiu-ying, H. *An Enumeration of Chinese Materia Medica.* Rev. ed. Hong Kong: Chinese University Press.

Sheng Y., "Treatment of chemotherapy-induced leukopenia in a rat model with aqueous extract from *Uncaria tomentosa*." *Phytomedicine* 7, no. 2 (2000): 137–43.

Silverman, H.M. *The Pill Book.* Bantam Books, 1990.

Sobenin I.A., V.V. Pryanishnikov, et al. "The effects of time-released garlic powder tablets on multifunctional cardiovascular risk in patients with coronary artery disease." *Lipids in Health and Disease* 9 (2010): 119.

Starfield, B. "Is US Health Really the Best in the World?" *Journal of the American Medical Association* 284, no. 4 (2000): 483–85.

Stoyanchev, K., P. Petkov, et al. "Alternatives to the Use of Organic Trace Minerals (Fe, Se and Cu) in Prevention of Some Deficiency States in Pigs." *Trakia Journal of Sciences* 4, no. 3 (2006): 44–49.

Thomson Healthcare *PDR for Herbal Medicines.* Medical Economics Company, 1999.

Tierra, M. *The Way of Herbs.* Washington Square, 1980.

Tildesley N.T., D.O. Kennedy, et al. "*Salvia lavandulaefolia* (Spanish sage) enhances memory in healthy young volunteers." *Pharmacology, Biochemistry and Behavior* 75, no. 3 (2003): 669–74.

US Spice and Essential Trade. USDA circular series "FTEA." 1–92.

Visser, J. "Alternative Medicine in the Netherlands." In George Lewith and David Aldridge, eds, *Complementary Medicine and the European Community.* Saffron Walden: CW Daniel, 1991.

Werback, M. *Botanical Influences on Illness.* Third Line, 1994.

Williams, D.L., E.R. Sherwood, et al. "Therapeutic efficacy of glucan in a murine model of hepatic metastatic disease." *Hepatology* 5, no. 2 (1985): 198–206.

Winther K., K. Apel, G. Thamsborg. "A powder made from seeds and shells of a rose-hip subspecies (*Rosa canina*) reduces symptoms of knee and hip osteoarthritis: a randomized, double-blind, placebo-controlled clinical trial." *Scandinavian Journal of Rheumatology* 34, no. 4 (2005): 302–08.

Wu, F.E., et al. "Two new cytotoxic monotetrahydrofuran Annonaceous acetogenins, annomuricins A and B, from the leaves of *Annona muricata*." *Journal of Natural Products* 58, no. 6 (1995): 830–36.

Index

About the Author

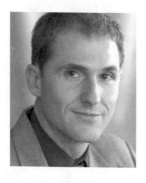

Tracy Gibbs, PhD, has an extensive background in pharmacognosy, the study of medicines derived from natural sources. Gibbs studied chemistry, hematology and botanical medicine in Japan where he received an honorary PhD from the Graduate School of Health Knowledge and Sciences (English name). He is a member of the International Iridology Practitioners Association, a board member in the International Health Food Research Foundation in Nagoya, Japan, and a member of the American Society of Pharmacognosy.

Gibbs has lectured worldwide on the clinical applications of herbal medicine. Gibbs operates an herbal medicine school in Japan and one in the United States where students can learn how to use herbs in everyday situations.

Gibbs has authored several books and booklets including *My Home Pharmacy, Phytonutrients: The Drugs of the Future* and *Your Blood Speaks*. Two of these books have been translated into Japanese-language editions.

Additionally, Gibbs is the owner and founder of Health Education Corporation, which specializes in nutritional blood evaluation, educational seminars, literature production and personal counseling. Gibbs is a co-owner and chief formulator for NutraNomics®, Inc., a Salt Lake City-based corporation that specializes in the research and development of nutritional supplements and herbal products.

Other Materials by Tracy Gibbs

Natural Products: Essential Resources for Human Survival
ISBN-13 978-981-270-498-6 or ISBN-10 981-270-498-1

Books Distributed by Woodland Publishing
Digestive Enzymes, 3rd Edition

Books Distributed by NutraNomics®
Your Blood Speaks
Blood Types and Nutrition

Check out these other top-selling Woodland Health Series booklets:

Ask for them by title or ISBN at your neighborhood bookstore or health food store. Call Woodland at (800) 777-BOOK for the store nearest you.

Each booklet is approximately 32 pages and priced at $4.95.

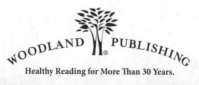

WOODLAND PUBLISHING

Healthy Reading for More Than 30 Years.